Exercises for Voice Therapy

Second Edition

Exercises for Voice Therapy

Second Edition

Edited by

Alison Behrman, PhD, CCC-SLP
John Haskell, EdD, CCC-SLP

PLURAL
PUBLISHING
INC.

SAN DIEGO
OXFORD
MELBOURNE

5521 Ruffin Road
San Diego, CA 92123

e-mail: info@pluralpublishing.com
Web site: http://www.pluralpublishing.com

Typeset in 10½/13 Garamond Book by Flanagan's Publishing Services, Inc.
Printed in the United States of America by McNaughton & Gunn

For permission to use material from this text, contact us by
Telephone: (866) 758-7251
Fax: (888) 758-7255
e-mail: permissions@pluralpublishing.com

Every attempt has been made to contact the copyright holders for material originally printed in another source. If any have been inadvertently overlooked, the publishers will gladly make the necessary arrangements at the first opportunity.

Library of Congress Cataloging-in-Publication Data

Exercises for voice therapy / Alison Behrman, editor ; John Haskell, editor.—2nd ed.
    p. ; cm.
Includes bibliographical references and index.
ISBN-13: 978-1-59756-530-1 (alk. paper)
ISBN-10: 1-59756-530-X (alk. paper)
I. Behrman, Alison. II. Haskell, John, 1937–
[DNLM: 1. Voice Disorders—therapy. 2. Exercise Therapy—methods. 3. Voice Training. WV 500]
RF510
616.85'560642–dc23
                     2013004663

Contents

Preface to Second Edition

Voice and voice disorders is a dynamic field of study. In the four years since the first edition of Exercises for Voice Therapy was published, we have witnessed (and, in many cases, participated in) a continued evolution of our field. New medical and scientific data and artistic innovations continue to broaden the breadth and depth of our practice. Our second edition bears witness to this vibrancy, with an expanded offering of treatment options for a wide variety of voice-related problems.

In this second edition, 17 voice therapists have joined the contributors' list, bringing fresh perspectives to the therapeutic process. Twenty-four new exercises are included for your consideration and exploration. We have retained the same overall chapter organization from the first edition, but almost every chapter includes expanded offerings. Three new exercises are designed specifically to address pediatric voice disorders. Three other new exercises focus upon vocal issues of transgendered clients. Additional approaches for paradoxical vocal fold dysfunction are presented in two new exercises. And the book now includes an exercise for clients with vocal tremor, as well as clients who routinely speak to larger audiences or conduct formal presentations. And you will find new offerings for vocal warm-ups and cool-downs, as well as additional exercises using a semi-occluded vocal tract, resonant voice therapy, integrating voice production with body movement, articulatory freedom, and vocal function exercises to facilitate improved glottal closure.

Once more, we wish to thank our contributors for the willingness to share their experience and creativity, and for their time and patience in the publication process. We are confident that you, our readers, will find this second edition an important assistant in your clinical practice, and that the book stimulates your own creativity as you continue to expand your voice therapy expertise. As always, we are happy to read your feedback and suggestions. Please feel free to email us, or to reach out to any of the contributors, whose contact information is provided, with questions or comments.

Preface to First Edition

The purpose of this book is to assist speech-language pathologists in developing treatment plans and session materials for clients—children and adults—with all types of voice disorders. Voice therapy is an emerging area of speech-language pathology, and voice therapists represent a small minority of speech-language pathologists. As a result, we have fewer resources that provide therapy materials. A wealth of information has been published regarding the nature of voice disorders and theoretical approaches to behavioral intervention, with case studies to illustrate conceptual approaches to different types of clients. But only a few published resources are available that provide the step-by-step process for achieving vocal change. Books on singing and acting technique may offer good information for developing new ideas for voice therapy. Conferences and workshops on voice disorders provide excellent opportunities to learn new approaches, observe our colleagues in demonstrations, discuss ideas, and receive inspiration. And e-mail is available for a quick note to a colleague, "Help, I've tried everything I know and she's still squeezing. Any ideas?" But no manual is available that represents a range of methods from a variety of clinical viewpoints for day-to-day planning of sessions.

So, we thought, why not broaden our circle of colleagues and share our ideas and suggestions in a format that can be accessed easily? Voice therapists around the world, working in a variety of clinical environments, have many great ideas, and we can all benefit from each others' experience and creativity. Thus, this book is motivated by our desire to help all of us share our therapy techniques so that we may all become better voice therapists.

Forty-eight exercises are included from 28 voice therapists. We use the term "exercise" to identify a set of tasks that has been organized into a cohesive activity for one or more therapeutic goals. From the Latin *exercitare*, to train, among its many meanings are "the act of bringing into play or realizing in action . . .

something performed or practiced in order to develop [or] improve" (Merriam-Webster, 2004). The difficulty levels of the exercises are varied. Some of them are suitable for novice voice therapists, whereas others require a greater depth of experience to be used most effectively. Similarly, voice clients will find some exercises more challenging than others. Although each exercise is presented in a consistent format, the different writing styles and topics reflect different theoretical approaches and training backgrounds of the contributors, thus adding richness to the book that would not otherwise have been possible. The exercises are organized into 10 chapters, each with a brief introduction. Terms that may not be familiar to all voice therapists are presented in bold type and defined in the Glossary. We elected not to organize the chapters by type of voice disorder. Instead, each chapter focuses on a parameter of the voice production system that may need to be addressed. We expect that these exercises will be used in a variety of ways, depending on the personal approach of each therapist and the needs of the individual client. Some of the exercises offer a basic framework for building an entire session, whereas others may fulfill a more specific need within a broader framework.

How did the contributors of this book come to be selected? In part, they selected themselves. We tried to contact many of the speech-language pathologists who have presented instructional clinical sessions at conferences or published articles on clinical methods in voice therapy. We called colleagues, and we asked colleagues to recommend other colleagues. We invited therapists to contribute one or more of their favorite exercises, to tell us from where the exercise originated, and how they modified the exercise from the original source to make it "their own." Most of the therapists we contacted agreed to participate. Some could not, for a variety of personal and professional reasons, and we are sorry to have missed their contributions.

Sharing therapy techniques is not easy. Voice therapy has been called both an art and a science, and many of the exercises may reflect more art than science. The evolving focus on the efficacy of voice therapy techniques may cause all of us to experience some reluctance to say "This exercise has worked with many of my clients and I'd like to share it with my colleagues." Therefore, when we share our therapies, we put our professional selves on display for everyone to judge. Fundamentally, we each ask ourselves "Am I a good voice therapist?" The evidence lies herein. Each voice therapist whose exercises are included in this book is an accomplished and thoughtful clinician who has been willing to share his or her ideas with you, the reader. Each therapist responded patiently through our editing process, answering our many questions and reviewing multiple changes, as we sought to clarify wording and intent. We are lucky indeed to be part of this community of voice therapists, and we owe a heartfelt "thank you" to each contributor.

We dedicate this book to our voice clients—past, present, and future—whom we hope to serve well. The process of creating a book is always a team effort. We thank our colleagues at Plural Publishing, a professional and knowledgeable team, particularly the wisdom and leadership of Dr. Sadanand Singh, the guidance of Judy Meyer, the highly talented production editor, Sandy Doyle, and Dr. Thomas Murry, whose advice and guidance are always insightful and on target. We thank Maury Aaseng, illustrator, who created the cover art and illustrations throughout the book. And we thank our colleagues, clients, and students on whom we tested these exercises.

A Word About the Accompanying CD

A CD accompanies this book, containing recordings of 25 of the exercises. The purpose of the CD is to provide an aural model for those exercises that may be difficult to interpret from the written text alone. Many of the exercises do not require a recording for comprehension of the exercise, while others may leave a reader uncertain as to how a task should sound without a recording for guidance. Those exercises included on the CD, many of which were recorded by the contributing author, have a CD icon next to the title. The table below lists the contents of the CD organized by chapter in which each corresponding written exercise can be found.

Contents of CD

Chapter 2

Track 1   Carroll, Vocal Cool Down

Track 2   LeBorgne Gentle Vocal Stretch and Contraction (Vocal Warm Up)

Chapter 4

Track 3   Gherson Trilled Carryover

Track 4   Klimek, Balancing Breath and Tone Through Advanced Trill/Flutter Tasks

Chapter 5

Track 5   Carroll, NG Sniff

Track 6   Haxer, Hyperfunctional Dysphonia

Track 7   Lader, Chant Talk

Track 8   Pinho, Spaghetti

Track 9   Schneider, Chant to Speak

Track 10   Schneider, Hum-Sigh with Chewing

Track 11   Yiu, Hong Kong Humming

Chapter 7

Track 12   Haskell, The Chewing Method

Track 13   Schneider, Tongue-Out Phonation

Track 14   Fava & Oliveira Tongue Teaser

Chapter 8

Track 15   Behrman, Calling the Text

Track 16   Klimek, Using Twang

Track 17   Ostrowski, Vocal Intensity Play

Track 18   Phyland, "Cooee" (The Aussie Bushman's Call)

Chapter 9

Track 19   Carroll, Vocal Fry to Modal

Track 20   Stemple Vocal Function Exercises

Track 21   Haxer, Hypofunctional Dysphonia

Track 22   Miller, Sharp Onset Vowel Sentences

Track 23   Miller, Up and Down Staccato

Chapter 11

Track 24   Block, Chant Your Pitch (Voice Feminization)

Track 25   Block, Count Big (Voice Masculinization)

Contributors

Julie Barkmeier-Kraemer, PhD, CCC-SLP
Professor, Voice, Speech, & Swallowing Center
Department of Otolaryngology
University of California, Davis
Davis, California
Chapter 11

Mara Behlau, PhD
Voice Specialist
Director, Centro de Estudos da Voz-CEV
Universidade Federal de São Paulo
São Paulo, Brazil
mbehlau@uol.com.br
Chapter 4

Alison Behrman, PhD, CCC-SLP
Department of Speech Communication Studies
Iona College
New Rochelle, New York
abehrman@iona.edu
All chapter introductions and Chapters 2, 3, 4, 8,
  and 11

Florence B. Blager, PhD, CCC-SLP
Professor Emeritus
Department of Otolaryngology
University of Colorado Health Science Center and
Department of Medicine
National Jewish Medical and Research Center
Denver, Colorado
blagerf@njc.org
Chapter 11

Christie Block, MA, MS, CCC-SLP
Speech-Language Pathologist
Private Practice
New York, NY
cblock@cblock.net
Chapter 11

Linda M. Carroll, PhD, CCC-SLP
Private Practice
424 West 49th Street, Suite 1
New York, New York
Senior Voice Research Scientist
Division of Otolaryngology
Department of Surgery
The Children's Hospital of Philadelphia
Philadelphia, Pennsylvania
lmcarrollphd@aol.com
Chapters 2, 3, 5, and 9

Karen Chan, PhD
Assistant Professor
Division of Speech & Hearing Sciences
The University of Hong Kong
Sai Ying Pun, Hong Kong
karencmk@hku.hk
Chapter 8

Philippe H. DeJonckere, MD, PhD
Professor
Catholic University of Leuven (B)
University of Lille II (F)
Emeritus Professor, Utrecht University (NL)
General Coordinator of the Scientific Council
Institute of Occupational Diseases, Brussels (B)
Belgium, The Netherlands
philippe.dejonckere@med.kuleuven.be
Chapter 2

Ellen Love Dungan, PhD, CCC-SLP
Private Practice—Voice and Speech Therapy
Consultant, Rye Country Day School
Larchmont, New York
voice5@aol.com
Chapters 3 and 10

Gaetano Fava, MS, CCC-SLP
Speech-Language Pathologist, Voice Specialist
Columbia University Medical Center
New York, New York
Atf9004@nyp.org
Chapter 7

Jackie L. Gartner-Schmidt, PhD, CCC-SLP
Associate Professor of Otolaryngology
University of Pittsburgh School of Medicine
Associate Director
Director of Speech-Language Pathology Services
University of Pittsburgh 1 Voice Center
Pittsburgh, Pennsylvania
gartnerschmidtj@upmc.edu
Chapters 3 and 11

Shirley Gherson, MA, CCC-SLP
Speech-Language Pathologist, Clinical Voice Specialist
Rusk Rehabilitation
NYU Langone Medical Center
New York, New York
shirley.gherson@nyumc.org
Chapters 4, 6, and 11

Edie R. Hapner, PhD, CCC-SLP
Associate Professor,
Director of Speech Language Pathology
Department of Otolaryngology Head and Neck
   Surgery
Emory University School of Medicine
Emory Voice Center
Atlanta, Georgia
ehapner@emory.edu
Chapter 2 and 9

John Haskell, EdD, CCC-SLP
New York, New York
haskellspeech@verizon.net
All chapter introductions and Chapters 3 and 7

Marc Haxer, MA, CCC-SLP
Clinical Speech-Language Pathologist Senior
Departments of Speech Pathology and
Otolaryngology/ Head and Neck Surgery
University of Michigan Health System

Ann Arbor, Michigan
Clinical Instructor
Department of Special Education
Eastern Michigan University
Ypsilanti, Michigan
haxer@med.umich.edu
Chapters 5 and 9

Rita Hersan, MS, CCC-SLP
Speech-Language Pathologist
Clinical Voice Specialist
University of Pittsburgh Voice Center
Pittsburgh, Pennsylvania
hersrg@upmc.edu
Chapter 10

Reinhardt Heuer, PhD, CCC-SLP
Professor Emeritus
Department of Communication Sciences and
   Disorders
College of Health Professions
Temple University
Philadelphia, Pennsylvania
reinhardt.heuer@temple.edu
Chapter 11

Michelle Horman, MA, CCC-SLP
Voice Pathologist
Singing Voice Specialist
Philadelphia Ear, Nose, and Throat Associates
Philadelphia, Pennsylvania
Chapter 6

Daniel Kayajian, MS, CCC-SLP
Co-Director, Voice modification Program for
   Transgendered Individuals at
The College of Saint Rose
Speech Pathologist specializing in Voice and
   Swallowing Disorders
Albany Medical Center Hospital
Department of Otolaryngology
Albany, New York
d7kaje@verizon.net
Chapter 11

Mary McDonald Klimek, MM, MS, CCC-SLP
Voice Consultant & Singing Voice Specialist

Lexington, Massachusetts
Vice President, Estill Voice International
Course Instructor, Estill Voice Training
mklimek@estillvoice.com
Chapters 4 and 8

Joan Lader, MA
Voice Consultant/Teacher
Private Practice
New York, New York
jlader@nyc.rr.com
Chapters 5 and 6

Wendy DeLeo LeBorgne, PhD, CCC-SLP
Voice Pathologist & Singing Voice Specialist
Clinical Director
Adjunct Assistant Professor, Cincinnati College
    Conservatory of Music
The Blaine Block Institute for Voice Analysis and
    Rehabilitation
The Professional Voice Center of Greater
    Cincinnati
Cincinnati, Ohio
wleborgne@soents.com
Chapter 2

Vicki Lewis, MA, CCC-SLP
Speech Pathologist
The Voice Care Center
The Ear, Nose, Throat, and Plastic Surgery
    Associates
Winter Park, Florida
vlewis@entorlando.com
Chapter 2

Juliana Litts, MA, CCC-SLP
Speech-Language Pathologist
Clinical Voice Specialist
University of Pittsburgh Voice Center
Pittsburgh, Pennsylvania
littsjk@upmc.edu
Chapter 11

Adam Lloyd, MM, MA, CCC-SLP
Speech-Language Pathologist
Singing Voice Specialist
Ear, Nose, Throat, and Plastic Surgery Associates

Winter Park, Florida
alloyd@entorlando.com
Chapter 2

Estella P.-M. Ma, PhD
Assistant Professor
Division of Speech and Hearing Sciences
Director, Voice Research Laboratory
Faculty of Education
The University of Hong Kong
Hong Kong
estella.ma@hku.hk
Chapter 7

Glaucya Madazio, PhD
Professor, Centro de Estudos da Voz-CEV
Universidade Federal de São Paulo
São Paulo, Brazil
glaumadazio@uol.com.br
Chapter 4

Reny Medrado, MS, CCC-SLP
São Paulo, Brazil
rsmedrado@uol.com.br
Chapter 9

Susan Miller, PhD, CCC-SLP
CEO, Voicetrainer, LLC
Washington, DC
Assistant Professor
Department of Otolaryngology–Head and Neck
    Surgery
Georgetown University Medical Center
Washington, DC
susan@voicetrainer.com
Chapters 3 and 9

Dominique Morsomme, SLT, PhD
Professor and Lecturer
University of Liège
Department of Psychology: Cognition and
    Behavior, Voice Unit
Voice Therapist, Ear, Nose, and Throat Department
University Hospital of Liège
Sart Tilman, Belgium
Dominique.morsomme@ulg.ac.be
Chapter 5

Thomas Murry, PhD, CCC-SLP
Department of Otolaryngology–Head & Neck
　Surgery
Weill Cornell Medical Center
Adjunct Professor of Biobehavioral Sciences
Teachers College, Columbia University
New York, New York
thm7001@med.cornell.edu
Chapter 11

Gisele Oliveira, PhD
Voice Specialist
Professor, Centro de Estudos da Voz-CEV
Sao Paulo, Brazil
gi_oliveira100@hotmail.com
Chapters 4 and 7

Rosemary Ostrowski, MM, MS, CCC-SLP
Voice and Singing Voice Therapist
Thomas Jefferson University Hospital
Private Practice, Voice Therapist/Voice Teacher
Philadelphia, Pennsylvania
rovoice@yahoo.com
Chapter 8

Ashley Paseman, MA, CCC-SLP
Speech-Language Pathologist
Vocal Pointe Private Practice
Syracuse, New York
vocalpointe@twcny.rr.com
Chapter 6

Brian E. Petty, MA, CCC-SLP
Speech Pathologist and Singing Voice Specialist
Emory Voice Center
Atlanta, Georgia
brian.petty@emoryhealthcare.org
Chapter 4

Debbie Phyland, MS
Speech Pathologist,
Voice Medicine Australia
Melbourne Voice Analysis Centre
Lecturer and Subject Coordinator,
La Trobe University
School of Human Communication Sciences

Victoria, Australia
d.phyland@latrobe.edu.au
Chapters 5 and 8

Jack Pickering, PhD, CCC-SLP
Professor of Communication Sciences and Disorders
College of Saint Rose
Speech-Language Pathologist
Capital Region ENT
Albany, New York
pickerij@strose.edu
Chapter 11

Sílvia Maria Rebelo Pinho, PhD, SLP
Director
INVOZ - Comunicação e Voz Profissional
São Paulo, Brazil
Voicesrp@uol.com.br
Chapters 5 and 9

Marci Daniels Rosenberg, MS, CCC
Speech Language Pathologist
Voice & Singing Specialist
Vocal Health Center
Departments of Speech Language Pathology &
　Otolaryngology
University of Michigan
Ann Arbor, Michigan
marcied@med.umich.edu
Chapter 4

Leah Ross-Kugler, MS, CCC-SLP
Voice Rehabilitation Specialist
Institute for Voice and Swallowing
Phelps Memorial Hospital
Sleepy Hollow, New York
Private Practice
Brooklyn, New York
Lrosskugler@gmail.com
Chapter 10

Bari Hoffman Ruddy, PhD, CCC-SLP
Associate Professor
Department of Communication Sciences and
　Disorders
University of Central Florida

Director,
The Voice Care Center
The Ear, Nose, Throat, and Plastic Surgery
    Associates
Winter Park, Florida
Bari.hoffmanruddy@ucf.edu
Chapter 2

Sarah L. Schneider, MS, CCC-SLP
Director Speech-Language Pathology Services
UCSF Voice and Swallowing Center
Department of Otolaryngology-Head and Neck
    Surgery
University of California-San Francisco
San Francisco, California
sarah.schneider@ucsfmedctr.org
Chapters 5 and 7

Martin L. Spencer, MA, CCC-SLP
Voice Pathology, Performance Specialist
The Voice Clinic at OhioENT
Columbus, Ohio
martin_spencer@ameritech.net
Chapters 6 and 11

Joseph Stemple, PhD, CCC-SLP, ASHAF
Professor
Division of Communication Sciences and
    Disorders
University of Kentucky
Lexington, Kentucky
jcstem2@email.uky.edu
Chapter 9

Shirley Tennyson, MA, EdM, CCC-SLP
Care of the Professional Voice
Singing Voice Specialist
Private Practice
New York, New York

shirley.tennyson@gmail.com
Chapter 2

Judith Maige Wingate, PhD, CCC-SLP
Director of Clinical Education
Clinical Associate Professor
University of Florida
Gainesville, Florida
wingate@ufl.edu
Chapter 10

Jessica Wolf
The Art of Breathing
New York, New York
jessica@jessicawolf.net
Chapter 6

Edwin M-L Yiu, PhD
Professor
Division of Speech and Hearing Sciences
Co-Director, Voice Research Laboratory
Faculty of Education
The University of Hong Kong
Hong Kong
eyiu@hku.hk
Chapters 5 and 11

Aaron Ziegler, MA, CCC-SLP
Acting Assistant Professor
Communication Sciences and Disorders
John A. Burns School of Medicine
University of Hawaii at Manoa
Honolulu, Hawaii
Ph.D. Candidate
Communication Sciences and Disorders
University of Pittsburgh
Pittsburgh, Pennsylvania
asz@hawaii.edu
Chapter 9

Chapter 1

THE PRACTICE OF VOICE THERAPY

"I'm Seeing a Case of Nodules . . ."

No matter how much experience we gather in voice therapy, we each recall our early clinical introduction. "Can I use this exercise with nodules?" "What do I do with presbyphonia?" Each question was asked with a certain sense of alarm, as though a different "recipe" for therapy was required for each diagnosis. With experience, we came to realize that the commonalities across voice therapy patients are very much greater than the differences. The biomechanics of voice production is the glue that binds our clients together. And that commonality of experience helps build our clinical expertise, for we can say, "I have seen this problem before, and these are some of the types of approaches that have worked for others with this problem." If we had to start from the very beginning with each voice therapy client, our work would be difficult, indeed. Yet at the same time, each client brings unique features to the therapy—laryngeal pathology, anxieties, vocal needs, to name a few—requiring us to make choices in our therapies regarding how best to serve their needs.

Making Choices

Voice therapy is, to a great extent, about making choices. We help our clients to increase the number of vocal choices available to them. Pitch and loudness can be used with greater flexibility. Breath support can be adapted to meet the demands of the phrase. Resonance can be altered to achieve a different internal sensation for the speaker, and a different voice quality for the listener. Often, our clients are not aware that vocal choices are available to them ("I've always run out of breath easily when I talk"), or they don't know how to access those choices ("I try to talk louder but it's just so tiring"). The voice therapist, therefore, has the challenge and responsibility to shape the client's conceptual approach to voice, as well as the client's vocal behaviors, so that the client becomes self-reliant and is able to make healthy and useful vocal choices.

Our therapeutic decision-making process also includes selection of vocal tasks, or exercises, of course, and this book is designed to facilitate that process. But prior to task selection, we choose the portion of the voice production system to which we want to direct our efforts. We may elect to focus on the subsystem of voice production that we believe is *driving* the problem. ("If he'd use better speech-breathing support, so many of his other symptoms would be minimized.") We may also choose to focus on a specific feature, or component, of the voice production system. For example, for a client with muscle tension dysphonia, we might select exercises that address reduction in tension of the tongue by changing its posture and movements. Another client with tongue tension might benefit from a focus on thoracic tension, which appears to be limiting breath support, and, in turn, triggering articulatory tension. Alternatively, we might choose to take a more holistic approach. The word holistic is defined as "relating to or concerned with . . . complete systems rather than with the analysis of, treatment, or dissection into parts" (Merriam-Webster, 2004). The holistic approach reaches across many components at once, and may involve a single gesture, or behavioral focus, that affects the entire system, for example, chewing or lip buzzes.

We may also make decisions that consider the client's readiness to participate in a treatment approach. We may select a focus that is easiest for the client to address, even if we believe that other factors are the "major" cause of the voice problem. ("I don't think she's ready to address the psychodynamic issues yet, so we're working on the hyperfunction through freeing posture and upper body movements.") We make these decisions because we know that the voice production system is a complex interplay of many factors, each exerting control on the other, and we can't address everything in each session.

On several occasions since the publication of the first edition of this book, we, as co-editors, were asked, "What exercises do you recommend for a patient with a polyp (or nodules)?" This is not an easy question and, here again, we are faced with a number of considerations and choices: disorder variables (onset, etiology, severity, etc.), client variables (age, use of voice, motivation, etc.), financial and/or time considerations, and, finally, clinician variables (knowledge, experience, comfort level with different types of methods).

We noted above the contrast between holistic and segmental frameworks for voice therapy. Holistic approaches are "therapies that strive to balance the three subsystems of voice production (respiratory, phonatory, resonatory) at once, as opposed to working directly on single voice components (segmental framework)" (Stemple et al., 2010). Perhaps, as a general rule, a therapist with limited voice therapy experience might feel more comfortable with a segmental framework (e.g., breath control, glottal onset, pitch and loudness variability). With more experience, the therapist might try a holistic approach, such as resonance voice therapy or the chewing method. Ultimately, we are always asking and choosing, "What's suitable for the patient, and what's suitable for me as the therapist?"

Integrating the Exercises into the Voice Therapy

Decision-making occurs throughout the therapeutic process: the identification and analysis of a problem, the establishment of goals, and the choice of therapeutic approach and procedures, with accompanying methods of reinforcement and transfer. Most of the exercises contained in this book are procedures to be included within a broader therapeutic approach, and are designed to be used in a hierarchy of training stimuli, from easiest to most difficult. (See Table 1–1 for an example of a training hierarchy.) In the early stages, a relatively lower or easier level of practice may be constructed using stimuli that facilitate the behavioral target. For example, we might use "um-hum" to achieve forward oral resonance. This type of facilitative training utterance is often referred to as a "trigger." Other stimuli or triggers within the training hierarchy may include imagery or the use of visual or tactile sensory modalities. As the target behavior emerges, these stimuli become cues and reinforcement.

As the client's responses become more secure, cues and feedback may be faded gradually as the exercise is applied to more difficult stimuli. The therapist may also elect to move the client up and down the hierarchy of stimuli. For example, after introducing and practicing the target, it may be elicited in short conversation for a few minutes, with lesser accuracy of production accepted. This approach may help a client understand how the new voice production can be incorporated into actual speech. ("I can't really do it right now, but I can see how it might work as I get better at it.") It may also provide an opportunity to try out the new target behavior within the context of changes in articulation and breath pressure, as well as variations in pitch, loudness, and rhythm that are an inherent part of conversation.

Negative practice may be used at any step of the way within the training hierarchy. "Can you do it the old way now, so that it feels effortful and uncomfortable?" followed by "That sounded like it was a lot of work to produce. Now can you say it the new way so that it is easy and comfortable?" The contrast between incorrect and correct productions may enable clients to gain confidence in self-correction of errors, thereby exerting control over the choices they make about their voice production. Thus, as clients progress

Table 1–1. A Hierarchy of Stimuli for Training and Practice

Levels of difficulty based on sound, linguistic, and cognitive loads

  Sustained sound (vowel, nasal, or other continuant)

  Sound combinations (mono- through multisyllabic)

  Rote speech (counting, days of the week)

  Repetition of a verbally presented model

  Reading

  Simplified conversation on a mundane topic
      "List the steps in making a turkey sandwich."
      "Describe what you see in this room."
      "Tell me how you traveled to this therapy session today."

  Conversations using personally familiar material
      "Pretend I am one of your sales clients and describe your product."
      "Describe the homework assignment as you would to your students."

  Conversation about novel or emotionally laden content

Blending levels

  Read or speak a phrase using only the vowels

  Chant a phrase to remove voice onsets and offsets and pitch changes

  Recite the alphabet using exaggerated prosody to tell a story or convey an emotion

  Precede a challenging utterance with a foundational phrase or trigger

  Embed facilitative words or phrases into lengthier utterances

through stages of training stimuli, with constant decision-making about the stimuli and reinforcement, they learn to become their own voice therapists.

Using New Vocal Skills Outside the Therapy Room

We make choices in voice therapy about facilitating transfer of new vocal behaviors from the therapy session to life outside the session. This process is no simple matter and it requires some strategizing on our part.

Part of the transfer process, of course, includes practice within naturalistic contexts. Clients are asked to integrate, in a hierarchic manner, a specific technique into communicative activities of daily living. ("Use the increased breath support when taking on the telephone at work.") But the transfer process also includes practice of drills, often assigned for a given duration and/or number of times per day, in a given order and with specific utterances. ("Do the lip buzzes, the chanted phrases, and then the articulation exercise for five minutes four times daily.") It is hoped that the act of focused practice session will help to remind clients about the techniques and strategies that are developed during the therapy sessions. It is hypothesized that the drills improve the clients' abilities to produce the target motor skills, and increase the likelihood the skills will carry over into subsequent talking, at least for a short time. And it is hoped that increasing the frequency with which clients think about new voice production behaviors helps them to change their vocal behaviors.

To help clients transition from therapy room to "real life," clients may also be asked simply to *think* about or be aware of target vocal behaviors within a communicative context. ("In class, observe your posture and head positions as you talk to the students.") Often, when a client is asked to produce a series of utterances and simply to pay attention to a variable (lip movement, for example), the client does make some motor adjustments, despite the therapist's urging to "not change anything, just observe." An example (true story) will illustrate this point. A therapy session is started with the query "How did your homework practice go this week?" The client reports that he did not have an opportunity to practice at all because the week had been so hectic. Yet in the next breath, he reports that the exercises are helping his voice tremendously. Further discussion revealed that he *thought* about the exercises frequently and he considered that this process resulted in increased awareness of his vocal targets, which helped him to achieve those targets. The improvement in his voice during the therapy session seemed to support his statement. Although we might prefer him to think about *and* to perform the exercises, the anecdote does remind us that we may not always know how the client is performing a task, or how the effect is achieved.

Some information can be conveyed to clients with relative speed, such as much of the standard vocal hygiene advice. And sometimes, a vocal exercise is a one-time event, used to instill awareness or facilitate a simple motor behavior. Other novel motor behaviors, such as how to achieve a forward oral resonance, for example, may require a slower and more complicated learning process across multiple sessions with home practice between sessions. Our clients can surprise us, however, in what they find easy or difficult to learn, and what facilitates or inhibits carryover. And, of course, it is these surprises that challenge us as voice therapists to forever remain flexible in our therapeutic approaches.

Leading Clinical Influences in Voice Therapy

As voice therapists, we owe much to a number of clinical leaders in our field, among them Moya Andrews, Arnold E. Aronson, Daniel R. Boone, Janina K. Casper, Lorraine O. Ramig, Nelson Roy, Joseph Stemple, and Katherine Verdolini. Their collective works provide the cornerstone of our voice therapy. Andrews' (2002) expertise in pediatric voice therapy has guided many therapists in working with children and adolescents with voice problems. Although many features of voice therapy are similar across all ages of our clients, different types of voice disorders are more prevalent at specific ages, and the goals and therapeutic approaches are different depending on the age of the client.

Through their teachings and writings, Aronson (1981) and Boone (2004) have provided considerable direction in regard to theoretical and practical approaches to voice therapy. One of the many practical concepts that Boone has addressed, for example, is use of facilitating techniques. How can we alter our clients' biomechanics quickly and easily so that their voices are more efficient, more easily produced, more pleasing in vocal quality, and better meet their communicative needs? In our evaluation and therapy, we seek to find facilitative techniques—triggers that help our clients move toward target vocal behaviors. Those facilitative techniques are then shaped into manners of voice production that serve our clients best.

Casper (Colton, Casper, & Leonard, 2006) has explored the connection between therapeutic techniques and the pathophysiology of vocal fold vibration, as observed through videolaryngeal stroboscopy. She guides us in the repair of damaged voices through *confidential voice*, in which the client uses a soft and breathy speaking voice to reduce the force of vocal fold contact. Ramig (Ramig, Fox, & Sapir, 2004) has developed and researched Lee Silverman Voice Therapy, a programmatic therapy for clients with Parkinson's disease. Her program offers a novel and proven approach for those of our clients with a specific neurologic disease. Roy (Roy, Bless, Heisey, & Ford, 1997), through his work with digital laryngeal manipulation, has helped us to learn how to use our hands to reposition the larynx, thereby eliciting more coordinated and efficient voice production from our clients who demonstrate muscle tension dysphonia. Stemple's Vocal Function Exercises (2000), a program of vocal "stretching" exercises, gives our clients a hierarchical set of phonatory tasks that addresses a variety of symptoms by targeting vocal flexibility and stamina. And Verdolini's development and research of the Lessac-Madsen Resonant Voice Therapy program (Verdolini, Druker, Palmer, & Samawi, 1998) offers us an approach that can be used with a wide range of clients experiencing vocal problems.

Numerous other outstanding clinicians have helped to lead our clinical work forward. And, certainly, each of us has had our own teachers, clinical supervisors, colleagues, and mentors who have provided training, guidance, and new ideas for our clinical practices. The exercises contained within this book draw on the expertise of all of these individuals, adding new pieces, reshaping others, but always with the greatest respect for their origins.

Seeking Evidence for Our Therapeutic Exercises

The exercises contained in this book are largely unproven. The current interest in evidence-based therapy is substantial and continues to grow. And whereas many voice scientists and therapists call for objective data to support the efficacy of voice therapy, few are willing or able to provide the data. Designing and conducting clinical trials that appropriately test the outcomes and efficacy of our therapies is extraordinarily difficult. Funding, subject accrual, a multitude of design factors with the potential to confound our ability to test clinical hypotheses, and lack of rigorous and objective outcome measures are among the most significant impediments to obtaining evidence of efficacy. And so, what are we to do in our therapies? At one end of the continuum, we could use only those techniques that have been proven to work and for which the underlying biomechanical changes are certain. But then we would have little to offer our clients. At the opposite extreme, we could rely wholly on our clinical experience and assert confidently to our clients that the exercises we use will most certainly address their vocal problems, providing of course that our clients are diligent in their practice and adhere to all therapeutic recommendations. In this vein, we could proceed to explain, with clarity and assurance, the biomechanisms by which our exercises are effecting the desired vocal change. But unfortunately, if we took that approach, then surely we would be misleading our clients. For no matter how certain we are that our clinical judgments are accurate, often our therapeutic outcomes are not what they appear to be. Perhaps an exercise may work, but not for the reasons that we think. Or perhaps the client is doing something different from what we believe to be occurring. Or perhaps we have been swayed by current dogma and our perception of events is biased.

And so we ask again, given the paucity of efficacy data, what are we to do in our therapies? The imperfect answer lies somewhere along the continuum between the extremes, of course. We can be cautious in our hypotheses of the biomechanical factors that drive our clients' voice problems, and the ways in which our exercises address those factors. We can qualify our discussions with clients, using words like *beliefs*, *hypotheses*, and *assumptions*. We can question our own beliefs about what is true and false, and continue to read the current literature in our own and related fields. We can refuse to become complacent. We can share our ideas, approaches, and exercises in an effort to help each other think along different pathways, explore new ideas, and continue to grow and improve, benefiting ourselves, our clients, and our field.

Chapter 2

BEFORE AND AFTER

In this section, we draw your attention to three issues that are, in a fashion, preparatory to other activities (the *before* part) or a result of an event or situation (the *after* part). We include here guidance for the voice evaluation, relative voice rest after vocal fold trauma, and cool-down exercises after heavy voice use.

In an evaluation, one of the goals is to determine the degree to which the voice problem can be altered through behavioral means. Not only do our evaluative tasks provide information about the nature and severity of the voice problem, but as DeJonckere highlights in *Vocal Plasticity*, they also give an indication of what types of facilitating techniques may yield rapid positive change. A voice with plasticity is able to be shaped quickly toward a more desirable voice: that is, the voice is *stimulable* for change. The change may be small or large, but it usually signals that *some* change through behavioral intervention is possible. It is then for us, as therapists, to further shape the change into a technique that is functional for the client in natural speech activities.

Also in regard to assessment, Hapner's Ruler Exercise provides a method of evaluating the client's potential for change—in other words, the likelihood of compliance. And similar to Vocal Plasticity, Ruler Exercise also helps guide the therapist in treatment planning.

Before demanding voice use, a gentle, progressive series of vocal tasks is often used to warm up the vocal mechanism, similar to the warm-up exercises used by athletes prior to intense physical activity. Three exercises are offered here: LeBorgne's Gentle Vocal Stretch and Contraction and Tennyson's Throat Openers both help the client prepare for strenuous talking with vocal maneuvers, whereas Tennyson's Laryngeal Massage combines a hands-on technique with vocalizing.

Therapeutic management of vocal fold trauma may be part of a "before" and an "after" situation. We must help the client manage the trauma, perhaps arising from stressful vocal demands or laryngeal surgery, after it has occurred. Before we work on many of therapy goals, however, the mucosa must reach some stage of healing. Relative voice rest, a substantial reduction in talking, is often part of the initial management plan used after the trauma has occurred, to help promote mucosal repair, and in other cases before an episode of demanding voice use, to help prevent trauma. Typically, in relative voice rest we amend not only the amount or duration of talking but also the manner in which our clients speak. Behrman's *Light and Easy Talking* is a temporary manner of speaking that may help prevent or repair vocal fold trauma. It offers an expansion to the traditional soft and breathy target of Casper's "confidential voice," adding guidance for breathing, pitch control, and articulatory movements, to promote greater vocal choices for the client and to lay the groundwork for a well-supported, resonant voice as the vocal folds heal.

After demanding voice use, many professional voice users routinely use a cool-down routine (sometimes referred to as vocal "warm-downs"). It is usually a short routine of gentle vocalizing, as in "cooing" the /u/ vowel (as in coo), relaxed humming, talking lightly in a falsetto voice, and massage of the neck, throat, and lower face. Warm-downs may help release excessive muscle tension that may accumulate during loud or extended talking. We can use the analogy to athletes, in whom muscle cramping and strain can occur after demanding activities if the muscles are not stretched in a cool-down routine. Both Carroll's *Vocal Cool-Down* and Hoffman Ruddy's *Vocal Cool-Down* adapt singing exercises to the speaking voice, using downward pitch glides to help the vocal folds slacken after demanding voice use. After trying out these exercises, you might want to explore other exercises in this book to help your client "disengage" from demanding voice use. Singers, for example, often cool down their voices by reversing their warm-up routine, and making it shorter, softer, and lighter in vocal quality.

Vocal Plasticity

P. H. DeJonckere

Purposes

- To evaluate the nature of the client's voice disorder.
- To assess the degree to which the client can modify voice production.

Origin

This approach is drawn from many years' experience working with individuals with various types of voice disorders. Our center has conducted research in this area and found that, to some extent, outcome of functional therapy can be predicted by early vocal plasticity (DeJonckere, 1998; DeJonckere & Lebacq, 2001; DeJonckere & Wieneke, 2001; Martens, Versnel, & DeJonckere, 2007).

Overview

Plasticity of voice quality is the degree of improvement in deviant voice quality that can be achieved nearly instantly by changing certain basic parameters: posture, articulation and resonance, breathing, laryngeal position, precervical muscle tension, and auditory feedback. This exercise guides the clinician to investigate vocal plasticity during the voice evaluation. These procedures, which are found to facilitate rapid improvement, are then used during the subsequent therapy sessions in a hierarchy of speech contexts and progressively generalized to similar (or less assisted) voicing situations. The treatment ends with a habituation or integration process to achieve permanent change in the voice.

Note: Perceptual assessment of change in vocal quality as a result of probing vocal plasticity is the primary method of evaluation of outcome of this exercise. However, instrumental measures, such as acoustic analysis and electroglottography, can be very useful for obtaining objective documentation of change in voice and for measuring features of voice production that are not readily apparent from perceptual assessment alone.

The Exercise

1. Try changing one or more of the following parameters, with the goal of eliciting rapid improvement in vocal quality. Proceed in stepwise fashion, trying out each manipulation, and assess the degree of improvement in voice quality.

   Posture: Adjust the position of the shoulders and the head, including flexion or rotation, to realign asymmetry or imbalance. Phonate during isometric activation of neck extensors (against resistance) in order to relax the neck flexors.

   Breathing Mechanics: Initiate speech at a higher lung volume. Alter the amount of air used during speech, first using a bit more, then a bit less. Check to see if the air is flowing continuously throughout the phrase or held back.

   Laryngeal Position: Manually reposition the larynx. While producing voice, gently pull down on the larynx to lower it. Then, gently push the larynx back slightly in the neck while phonating. Finally, gently squeeze the larynx (compress it laterally) while phonating. Lower the larynx to phonate with a wide open mouth and active tongue depression (a dark /ɑ/). In this posture, the larynx should lower.

   Loudness: Increase the loudness level at which you speak. Louder speech may eliminate voice breaks at phonation onset or offset (including glottal fry), or may reduce excessive turbulent air escape. Alternatively, try decreasing the loudness level during speaking, which may help facilitate a greater sense of ease of phonation.

   Articulation and Resonance: Hum gently before speaking a phrase. Sustain vowels, such as /i/ and /u/, which create a partial occlusion in the mouth and can facilitate improved voice quality. Try increasing the range of motion of the lips, tongue, and mandible while speaking.

   Auditory Control: Induce a change in loudness, pitch, or quality by putting on headphones through which white noise is played (the Lombard-Tarneaud effect). Using sustained vowel or connected speech, the change in internal auditory feedback may elicit an altered coordination of musculature used to produce voice.

2. Once it is discovered that altering a specific parameter yields improved voice quality, practice it repeatedly until the behavior is stable and improved voice quality is achieved consistently.

3. Now begin to generalize the behavior to other speech conditions, including:

- Vowels with different degrees of openness
- Varying pitch and loudness
- Consonants
- Rote speech
- Reading
- Spontaneous speech

4. As success with generalization is achieved, gradually fade the condition that induced the change when such condition cannot be habituated in normal conversation. For example, speaking more loudly or using greater lung volume on initiation of phonation can be maintained in routine speaking situations. However, manual manipulation of the position of the larynx must be faded.

Ruler Exercise

Edie Hapner

Purposes

- To engage the client in the therapy process
- To identify the client's perceived barriers to changing vocal behavior
- To define the strategies needed to assist the client through vocal behavior change.

Origin

The ruler exercise is not a therapy technique but rather a method of quickly assessing how the client feels about voice therapy and their ability to complete voice therapy successfully. The ruler exercise was developed by Prochaska, Norcross, and DiClemente (1994) as a method to assess a person's confidence and commitment to making a health behavior change. It is a fundamental part of the counseling technique called Motivational Interviewing (MI) developed by Miller and Rollnick (1991) but can be used in a therapy process with or without MI counseling.

Overview

I use the Ruler Exercise during my initial contact with clients to determine their confidence that voice therapy is a useful method to address the voice problem. If they lack the confidence in therapy from the beginning, no shows, homework not completed, and drop-outs may follow. The ruler exercise takes only a few minutes and helps me identify gaps in information, or a lack in self-confidence, and then address those gaps up front. It also allows me to address the commitment to attending and completing voice therapy. If clients are concerned that voice therapy is just one more thing on their already busy schedule, or if they are not sure they can get off work to attend voice therapy, the ruler exercise lets me know this and helps clients address these commitment concerns. I often use the ruler exercise at the end of a therapy session after giving homework to determine the confidence and commitment to completing the homework assignments.

COMMITMENT

> *This box is 5 inches long and can be divided into 10 ½-inch equally spaced and numbered tabs 1 to 10. You can also use a 10-cm ruler like the ASHA SIG3 CAPE-V rulers. Put the words confidence and commitment in boxes above and below the ruler.*

COMMITMENT

The Exercise

1. Place the 10-point ruler in front of the client (a woman, for example). Ask her any one of these questions as appropriate to determine commitment to change.

   "On a scale of 1 to 10, how convinced are you that making changes in the way you use your voice will make a difference in your voice quality (or your loudness, or your effort, or your pain, whatever the primary problem)?"

2. After she chooses a number, ask her the following question:

   "You chose _____, why aren't you a _____? (Note, start with one number higher than what she chose. For example, if she chose 4, ask her why it is not a 5).

   This question allows clients to verbalize why they are not choosing a higher number. Perhaps it is because they have had therapy before and it was not successful or they know someone who has had therapy and it was not successful. This will open up the opportunity to discuss how your therapy is different from the prior therapy or why a pill or surgery isn't the best first choice, if they say they just wanted a medical intervention.

3. Then ask the client to respond to this question:

   You said _____, why aren't you a _____? (Note, start with one number lower than what she chose. For example, if she chose 4, ask her why she is not a 3.)

This exercise allows clients to explain to you why they are more committed to the process. Sometimes their self-talk is all they need to increase their commitment to the behavior change and voice therapy. Be sure to ask this question second so that clients end on a high note, convincing you they are committed.

4. Repeat the process of placing the ruler in front of the client and this time ask:

   "On a scale of 1 to 10, how confident are you that you can make a change with your voice?"

5. After a number is chosen, ask the client the following questions:

   "You chose _____, why aren't you a _____? (Note, start with one number higher than what the client chose. For example, if she chose 4, ask her why she is not a 5.)

   This will open up the opportunity to discuss the barriers the client may perceive that hinder her ability to make a change.

6. Then ask the client to respond to this question:

   You said _____, why aren't you a _____? (Note, start with one number lower than what was chosen.)

   Be sure to ask this question second so that the client ends on a high note convincing you she is confident she can make a change.

Motivational Interviewing (MI) uses the responses to these questions to guide you in how to talk to the client about making a change. If you want to read more about MI, review Miller and Rollnick's seminal book entitled: *Motivational Interviewing: Preparing People for Change*, Second Edition, 2002 or Rollnick, Mason, and Butler's book entitled: *Health Behavior Change, A Guide for the Practitioner*, 1999. Also, Behrman wrote a great article on MI and its use in voice therapy (Behrman, 2006).

Gentle Vocal Stretch and Contraction (Vocal Warm-Up)

Wendy D. LeBorgne

Purposes

- To warm up the voice prior to more intense vocalization following a "cold" state
- To coordinate respiration, phonation, resonance, and intensity.

Origin

Based on theories of exercise physiology, traditional acting voice training, and voice therapy techniques, these exercises are designed to be used by actors as a warm-up before beginning more intense vocalization. A professional dancer likely would not get out of bed and immediately do a split without some gentle stretching first. And an actor would not begin a rehearsal or performance without a vocal warm-up. Similarly, people who use their voices intensively, such as teachers, should warm up their voices to prepare their vocal mechanism for more intense use.

Overview

This three-part speaking voice warm-up begins with a general coordination of the respiratory, phonatory, and resonatory systems. The client then warms up the lower and upper parts of pitch and loudness ranges, moving into speech production. In the first exercise, Coordinated Voice Production, the client begins a relaxed inspiratory/expiratory pattern, coordinating gentle phonation in the middle part of the vocal range. In the second exercise, Pitch Variation/ Inflection, the client explores the lower and higher parts of the pitch range with short phrases. The third exercise, Intensity, provides the client with the opportunity to maximize and minimize vocal intensity, coordinating breath, sound, and characterization. The warm-up should take approximately 3 to 5 minutes.

The Exercise

Part I. Coordinated Voice Production

1. Inhale to a comfortable lung volume (do not overinflate, as you are only going to speak for a 7- to 10-second utterance). As you inhale, maintain awareness of your respiratory expansion, including the thorax and abdomen. Imagine you are smelling something good, for example, brownies, chocolate chip cookies, or a bouquet of flowers.

2. Following gentle inhalation, generate 4 or 5 speech-inflected syllables in a comfortable speaking range using one of the following: lip buzz-/m/-vowel or tongue trill-/n/-vowel. (Listen to the accompanying recording.) Pay attention to precise and coordinated onset, with a seamless transition from the buzz or trill into the /m/ or /n/. Visualize a magician pulling scarves out of his sleeve. Your breath and sound production should feel smooth and continuous like the scarves. Envision that the sound begins with breath and ends with vibration. There should be a seamless production between each repeated syllable with no detection of voice breaks.

Part II. Pitch Variation/Inflection

1. Explore pitch variation through inflected 5-syllable phrases. Begin in the comfortable part of your speaking voice. (Shorter or longer phrases may be used, or lines from a working script, depending on the needs of the actor.) Continue to breathe, as above, but before you say each phrase, inhale only as deeply as necessary to say the phrase.

2. Repeat each phrase three times. With each repetition, use a different inflection pattern, as if you want to communicate something different with each inflection.

   Five-Syllable Practice Phrase (examples). (Listen to the accompanying recording.)

   I am so very sad.

   You are a bad dog.

   Why did you call me?

   I love you so much.

   You have a nice house.

Part III. Intensity

1. In order to warm up vocal intensity, explore variations from a whisper to a yell. However, maximum intensity is *not* advised

in this exercise. You should use neutral syllables from Part I, the five-syllable phrases in Part II, or short phrases of your choosing.

2. Say each of the following phrases a total of three times with three different intentions and vocal intensity, for example, soft, whisper, conversational, shout, and so forth.

Five-syllable Practice Phrases (examples). (Listen to the accompanying recording.)

Please eat more apples.

You are my best friend.

The sun is setting.

One, two, three, four, five.

He/she has had enough.

Throat Openers

Shirley Tennyson

Purposes

- To warm up the voice
- To expand the pharynx by inhibiting throat constriction and laryngeal elevation
- To balance intrinsic laryngeal muscle activity by promoting thinning/stretching in balance with thickening/contracting functions of the vocal folds
- To prepare for resonance exercises.

Origin

My years of study with singing teacher Cornelius Reid taught me the value of "opening the throat" for singing. I have found it an invaluable concept for the speaking voice as well. I have borrowed from various voice therapy and singing exercises to develop this series of exercises to help reduce throat constriction in speaking.

Overview

Generally, I start with circumlaryngeal massage (see Laryngeal Self-Massage in this volume) to begin the process of unloading excessive vocal tract tension. Depending on the needs of the client, I will often introduce these throat openers as a way to expand the pharynx and release throat tension "from the inside." At times, I may choose to begin with resonance, but if a client has difficulty achieving the targeted tone focus, I find that reducing throat tension first has a positive effect on resonance. All the exercises are done with an exaggerated "yawny" stretch (the beginning part of a yawn). I explain to the client that this is not a way to speak, but, rather, the exaggeration helps one feel the contrast to constriction. It also inhibits the strong constrictor muscles that elevate and close the throat during swallowing, a position that is not ideal for speaking. The exercises should be done at a soft to moderate loudness level, except where indicated.

The Exercise

1. Yawn/Sigh. Yawn (or simulate a yawn) with a broad inhalation, and exhale with a sigh "hah" with lots of airflow and a breathy

sound. Then, repeat with "hoo" and "ho." Maintain the exaggerated open throat for each sound, so that it sounds like you're phonating on a yawn. Perform each sound once.

2. Owl Hoots. Start a broad yawn, and then make a soft, hollow sound, much like you think an owl would sound. (Men: Use falsetto if you can, as if you are imitating a woman.) Perform a set of three hoots three times.

3. The Prima Donna Yoo-Hoo. Call out at a moderate loudness and comfortable pitch with an open throat, as if you are trying to get someone's attention. The "yoo" is higher than the "hoo" (a minor third). (Men: Use falsetto if you can.) Perform this step three times.

4. Waterfalls. Say each of the following syllables once, initiating a yawn before each syllable: "hoo, ho, ha, hee." Start each syllable at a comfortable high pitch with soft-to-moderate loudness and glide down to a comfortable lower note, increasing the loudness as you descend.

5. Dips. Using the words *HOOP* and, later, *HOPE*, begin the release of the yawn as softly as possible on a comfortable high pitch. Then increase your loudness as you descend to a comfortable low pitch, and then swing into an upward glide at moderate loudness. Do each one three times. If you have difficulty reaching a solid low note in the dips, phonate at your lowest comfortable low note (no vocal fry) before starting the dip. It may then be easier to reach that low pitch in the dip.

6. Wolf Howl. Begin on a full *AH* in chest voice (your regular speaking pitch), and then flip into a wide, open throat (lips are rounded and protruded) and a higher pitch for OOOOOO-ooooooo, letting it trail off after 3 or 4 seconds. Make it sound eerie, spooky, and far away. For a great model, it can be helpful to go online and search on "Wolf Howl" and then listen to an audio recording of real wolves.

> Note that although a smooth connection between registers is desirable, a rough transition is permissible and the client can flip into the lower note. Creating a smooth transition between registers can be very difficult for some clients. Reassure them that it may take some practice to achieve this glide smoothly all the way through.

> It is helpful to begin by having the client attempt to allow a real yawn, if possible, and describe the feelings in the back of the throat (such as the soft palate lifting, the larynx descending, the throat widening, etc.). Clinicians should alert the clients to the possibility of hyperventilation with yawn exercises. Keep in mind that the purpose of the yawn, after the first few times, is to replicate the stretching rather than the intake of a lot of air. If the client cannot achieve a yawn, there are several ways to facilitate the maneuver (with thanks to my colleague Rachel Coleman for some of these suggestions):
>
> ■ Stretch the arms wide and take a deep breath through a wide open mouth as if you are very tired
> ■ Start by sighing, gradually making the sigh deeper until it begins to feel like a yawn
> ■ Visualizations, such as making room to put a large goose egg in the throat, creating a "cathedral" in your throat

■ Modeling the yawn yourself in hopes that your client will "catch it"
■ Gasping as if startled.

Eventually, even the most tense or inhibited person usually responds to these exercises by laughing and loosening up, which also helps lower the larynx.

Laryngeal Self-Massage

Shirley Tennyson

Purposes

- To warm up the voice before speaking.
- To rebalance muscles and restore voice quality after extended use of voice.
- To provide clients with techniques to manage vocal fatigue, throat tension, and throat discomfort.
- To give clients more confidence in their ability to help themselves improve.

Origin

This set of exercises is derived from the teachings of Nelson Roy, Jacob Lieberman, DO (from England), and Marina Gilman. In my years of working with people with voice disorders, I have found that one of the most effective techniques for anyone struggling to phonate with some kind of voice problem has been circumlaryngeal manipulation and laryngeal repositioning. After this treatment, most people walk out of the initial assessment session feeling reduced throat tension, greater ease in phonation, and improved voice quality, sometimes dramatically so. They often ask what they can do to keep this feeling or voice quality beyond the therapy session. Strangely enough, even when initial assessment of the perilaryngeal area does not reveal excessive tightness or tenderness, treatment with these techniques brings a degree of improvement in most clients and elicits comments that their voice feels better.

Overview

These techniques that I teach the client to use on his or her own are only a portion of a more extensive treatment. My in-office protocol takes about 15 to 20 minutes and includes the exercises explained here. The home version takes 5 to 10 minutes, depending on the needs of the client. I provide clients with a handout of instructions, mark the appropriate ones, and recommend they practice the entire protocol once in the morning (the shower is a great place to do them) and again in the evening, with mini-practices using favored procedures whenever needed throughout the day.

Note: While I'm performing the techniques, I usually wear gloves. (They need to fit snugly.) I have a model of the larynx in

One must be cautious with elderly patients or those with heart problems. Be careful to avoid working too closely to the carotid arteries on both sides of the neck at the same time, as these arteries provide the major blood supply to the brain. If the client experiences any dizziness or lightheadedness, immediately discontinue this entire technique.

It is helpful to try these techniques on yourself to experience the sounds and sensations that may result from the manipulations. You may feel or hear crackling sounds (crepitus) on the wiggles or be surprised by the change in phonation as you pull down on the larynx. Pitch and quality changes are typical. I ask the client to sustain the sound, but to allow the change to take place. I also urge the client to pull down slowly, listen, and feel when the quality improves, and continue that quality for a few seconds. Be prepared for giggles (sometimes shyness) and make it fun.

view and explain how the larynx is in a sling of muscles, what I'm doing, and why these techniques can help relieve excessive tension and improve comfort and voice quality. Some clients are naturally protective of their throats. I always give them a brief overview of what I'm about to do and ask their permission. I also ask them to tell me if they want me to stop at any time and to report any tenderness or discomfort. If a client is extremely tender or squeamish about the manipulation, I demonstrate how to do it on myself and ask the client to follow along, using a tolerable amount of pressure. Usually, after doing this at home for a week or so, the client will allow me to do my full protocol.

The Exercise

Try all the steps below, then choose the most effective one(s) for daily practice:

1. Circles. (Figures 2–1 through 2–4.) Put one hand at a time on the opposite side of the throat. Massage the entire throat beginning underneath your jaw with a circular motion, gradually moving down to the clavicle (collar bone). After massaging, pull your hand diagonally from the under the ear to the center so the larynx moves slightly to the opposite side. Then, use

Figure 2–1. Circles 1a. Left hand on right side.

Figure 2–2. Circles 1b. Right hand on left side.

Figure 2–3. Circles 2. Both hands simultaneously.

Figure 2–4. Circles 3. Thumb on one side and fingers on the other side.

both hands to massage the entire area. Finally, use one hand, fingers on one side and thumb on the other.

2. Stretches. (Figures 2–5 through 2–7.) Place two fingers of each hand under each ear (anterior to the sternocleidomastoid muscle). Pull down firmly and slowly. Repeat three to four times. Then, move to the sides of the larynx, and repeat. Finally, using one hand, grasp your larynx in front, and pull down firmly six to eight times.

3. Wiggles. (Figures 2–8 and 2–9.) Place three fingers of each hand on either side of your larynx. Push it from side to side. It should move freely without resistance. Small, "crackly" sounds are normal.

Figure 2–5. Stretch 1. **Figure 2–6.** Stretch 2.

Figure 2–7. Stretch 3.

Figure 2–8. Wiggles: Push to the right. **Figure 2–9.** Wiggles: Push to the left.

4. Stretches Plus Vowels. As you pull your larynx down firmly and slowly (as in Stretches above). Sustain each of the words below, one time each at a comfortable low pitch, with a medium loud voice:

> Who- - - - - - - - - - →
>
> Ho - - - - - - - - - - - →
>
> Ha - - - - - - - - - - - →
>
> He - - - - - - - - - - - →

Note that if the volume is too soft, the exercise is not as effective. However, you may not want to do these vocal exercises initially if you are severely hoarse: instead, you might try a hum.

5. Jiggle and Press. (Figure 2–10.) Sustain the words above as you push in and out with the side of the index finger in a gentle pulsing motion for three or four seconds, then press the hyoid 2 or 3 seconds. Do 2 or 3 sets of jiggle and press. Note that if you place the back of your hand under your jaw touching the area of the throat, it puts your index finger at the level of the hyoid bone.

6. Tongue Press. (Figure 2–11.) Press a thumb upward in the center at the juncture of your jaw and throat and feel the back of your tongue lift. Hold a steady, firm pressure for 20 to 60 seconds. When you slowly release the pressure, feel the openness in your throat.

Figure 2–10. Hand position for Jiggle and Press.　　**Figure 2–11.** Tongue Press.

Light and Easy Talking

Alison Behrman

Purpose

■ To promote healing of the vocal fold mucosa in cases of significant **phonotrauma**.

Origin

This approach derives from *confidential voice* developed by Dr. Janina Casper. My variation of that popular technique evolved over the years working with clients who were placed on restricted speaking by their laryngologist due to acute phonotrauma or in the early postoperative period. Confidential voice focuses on speaking softly with a breathy voice quality. I found that many clients who tried to use confidential voice were "too careful." They limited pitch range and restricted range of motion of their articulators as they "walked on eggshells" with their voices, and ended up increasing overall tension of the voice production system. In response to that excessive caution, I developed Light and Easy Talking, which emphasizes safe production of a free and *energized* voice.

Overview

Light and Easy Talking is a temporary* style of voice production that should be used in conjunction with partial (modified) voice rest. Light and Easy Talking promotes gentle vibration of the vocal folds with reduced medial contact. It is hypothesized (but unproven) that gentle vibration of the vocal fold mucosa may help promote movement of the byproducts of the inflammatory process out of the tissues. Gentle vibration may also help prevent buildup of mucus on the vocal fold surfaces, perhaps decreasing the urge to throat-clear. Light and Easy Talking is a quiet and safe but energized style of speaking, thus making it more practical for real-life communicative requirements than simply speaking very softly. And finally, the emphasis on breath support, vocal flexibility, and articulatory movement form the basis of efficient voice production, making it easy to extend Light and Easy Talking into a well-supported, resonant voice when the period of voice rest is completed and the vocal fold mucosa is healed.

---

*The duration is variable for each individual and is determined by the laryngologist, the voice therapist, and the client.

The Exercise

1. Use a soft-moderate loudness level. Do not whisper or speak too softly. Under your therapist's guidance, explore talking in a range of soft-to-moderate speaking levels until you can speak at the target level consistently and easily.
2. Use a mildly breathy voice quality. The goal is to use incomplete vocal fold contact and mildly increased airflow. With your therapist, explore different degrees of breathiness until you find a level that, with practice, becomes comfortable for you.
3. Use low (abdominal) breath support during speaking. Even a soft voice needs to be well supported. Good speech-breathing support is particularly important with a breathy voice in which vocal fold contact is incomplete and extra airflow is used.
4. Use a moderately "singsong" style of speaking. That is, use a wider variety of pitches (highs and lows) when speaking than you typically use.
5. Use increased movement of the articulators, particularly the tongue and the lips. The goal here is *not* to overarticulate or enunciate precisely. Too often, the effort of careful enunciation actually increases tension in the voice production system. Instead, practice increasing your attention to the movements of your lips, then to your tongue, and finally to your jaw as you speak. For example, during a rote speaking task, such as recitation of the months of the year, focus on lip movement as you say the first four months, then focus on tongue movement for the next four months, and finally focus on jaw movement as you say the last four months. The goal is to allow these articulators to move fully and freely during speaking.

Some people use the word "breathy" or "airy" to describe the target voice quality. Others (particularly performers) associate negative characteristics with those descriptors. In that case, it may help clients to think about their speech as being moderately cushioned on a bed of air. Use of a one-to-five scale can help the client find the appropriate level of softness and breathiness, Ask clients to identify the number on the breathiness or loudness scale that corresponds to the level at which they are talking. Then ask them if they can move up (or down) one or more numbers.

Many clients experience particular difficulty achieving a widened pitch contour. Sometimes it is confused with a *higher* pitch or louder voice. Or clients think they are using a very wide pitch range, when, in fact, they are not. To help your clients achieve a wider pitch contour, ask them to imagine that they are talking to a young child or a puppy. It can also be helpful to have clients purposely exaggerate the singsong feature. Then, during multiple repetitions of the same speech material, ask them to "dial down" the singsong just a little bit each time until they are using an appropriately widened pitch contour. (After practicing the highly exaggerated pitch style, a moderately widened pitch contour may not sound so strange to them.) During this process, it may be helpful for the client to record these exercises and then listen to the different levels of pitch exaggeration.

Often, when a speaker tries to talk quietly to protect the voice, the range of motion of the lips, jaw, and tongue are reduced, usually unintentionally, as part of the "walking on eggshells" approach to limiting movements of the speech production system. But, in fact, freedom of movement is very important in Light and Easy Talking. Low effort with free movement of the articulators serves two purposes. First, it may inhibit the buildup of tension and rigid posturing of the muscles of the neck and larynx, features that are counterproductive to healthy vocal fold vibration. Second, generous movements of the articulators may help focus the energy of the voice in the front of the oral cavity, facilitating improved oral resonance. This type of resonance may maximize the ability of the vocal tract to energize the voice.

Vocal Cool-Down

Linda M. Carroll

Purposes

- To relax the vocal musculature after heavy vocal use.
- To reduce vocal fry.
- To reduce vocal strain.

Origin

Many performers are trained to use cool-down exercises after a performance. I originally developed this exercise to assist transition from the singing to the speaking voice after strenuous performance demands. Professional voice users such as politicians, sales people, and classroom teachers, often use their voices in a manner akin to the professional singer. All professional voice users can be considered vocal athletes and they can all benefit from the use of cool-down exercises.

Overview

During this exercise, the vocal folds are gradually slackened and then required to adjust tension level during the short pitch "wiggle" on the last note. This exercise is done only in the mid- to lower part of the vocal range. However, it could be initiated in the upper part of the range. Many clients exhibit improved focus and consistency of the speaking voice following this exercise, with fewer episodes of vocal fry.

The Exercise

1. Produce a descending five-tone scale (beginning in mid-range) on /o/. Hold the lowest note for three seconds on /ɑ/ with a slight vocal pitch "wiggle." (Singers should use a two-tone trill.) Be sure to maintain the breath support through the wiggle.
2. Continue the descending five-tone scale a half-tone lower.
3. Continue in half-tone steps, until the voice reaches a comfortable point at the low end of the pitch range.

Vocal Cool-Down

Bari Hoffman Ruddy, Vicki Lewis, and Adam Lloyd

Purpose

- To release tension in the larynx and supraglottal articulators following intensive voice use.
- To minimize tension in the base of the tongue and other articulators to promote relaxed voice production.

Origin

The Boone and McFarlane (1988) *yawn-sigh* technique influenced the development of this vocal cool-down exercise. This exercise was also shaped by principles adapted from the practice of "vocal yoga," an emerging practice combining the strategies of voice therapy and principles of traditional yoga (Lyle, 2012). The emphasis is on general body posture and breath coordination prior to voice onset and during phonation. We have found the combination of vocal sighs and articulatory movements to be useful in reducing observed muscle tension and vocal strain after loud or prolonged vocal use.

Overview

After rigorous vocal activity, cooling down the voice may be helpful. Similar to athletes who cool down with gentle stretches after an athletic event, occupational voice users may elect to vocalize on a gentle and softly engaged hum gliding down in a relaxed manner. Use of sounds such as "la," "na," "ma," or "blah" may help reduce tension in the base of tongue and articulators. The focus of any type of relaxation or cool-down exercise is to promote coordination of respiration and phonation, reduce vocal strain and harshness, reduce tension of the articulators, and help prevent vocal injury. This exercise is also often utilized with singers to begin to establish voice production with minimal muscle tension in the tongue, base of tongue, and articulators.

The Exercise

1. Begin by taking in a relaxed breath, allowing the tongue and jaw to relax during inhalation. Then, using an easy onset, quickly

and gently articulate the syllable "blah," on a descending sigh. Repeat 3 to 4 times until voice production feels effortless, and strain or glottal fry is no longer heard.

2. Repeat step one, this time using the syllable "nee-ah" and then again using "lah." Remember to produce the syllables with a sigh-like vocal quality and to keep your articulators relaxed. Vocal fry should be avoided. At the end of each sigh, your voice quality should be slightly breathy. Repeat this exercise 3 to 4 times in an effortless manner.

Note: The exercise can also be used as a cool down for singers. In that case, each step should be repeated 3 to 4 times, descending a half-step with each repetition.

Chapter 3

TEACHING SPEECH-BREATHING SUPPORT

Speech-breathing is the regulation of breathing for voice and speech production. A substantial portion of our voice therapy time and effort is devoted toward management of speech breathing. Often, it is one of the first goals that we address in therapy, and with good reason. The airflow drives the vocal folds to vibrate. The air is resonated by the vocal tract, and the resulting emitted air pressure wave *is* the speech sound wave— the product of all of our work.

Many of our clients do not match the depth of inhalation with the length of the breath group (the number of syllables spoken on a single exhalation). Some use too little air, and others use too much air. Some appear to barely expand their thoracic cavity as they inhale, whereas others hold their breath and appear unwilling or unable to release it in a smooth and controlled manner while speaking. Our therapies focus on increasing our clients' awareness of breathing during speech production, and increasing our clients' choices regarding management of speech breathing. They learn that, although coordination of breathing with speech is essential for good voice production, many choices are available regarding how to best realize that coordination for an individual phrase.

Five exercises are included in this section. Behrman's *Why Don't You?* uses progressive-length sentences to help the client match the depth of breathing with the duration of the phrase and the expressiveness of the utterance. Carroll's *Breath Pacing* is particularly helpful for training the appropriate timing and duration of inhalation. She uses a counting task to limit the linguistic demand so that the client can focus on breathing mechanics. Dungan and Haskell, in *Breathing Awareness,* use a progression of tasks, from counting to simple phrases, progressing to more complex linguistic material. In that way, they help the client to expand his or her choices about breathing and spoken content. Gartner-Schmidt's *Flow Phonation* uses a visual cue, a tissue placed in front of the lips, to help clients use appropriate breath flow coordinated with vocal fold vibration. Miller's *Relaxed Heart-Mind Breathing* uses postures of yoga and mental imagery to help the client release mental and physical stress, particularly during anxiety-producing communicative events.

Although only five exercises are found in this chapter, speech-breathing is addressed throughout this book within many of the other exercises. For example, Schneider's *Tongue-Out Phonation* (Chapter 7) teaches the open-breath, a good preparation for any vocal exercise. Similarly, Paseman, in *I Like to Move It! Move It! Kinesthetically Speaking* (Chapter 6), provides a series of stretching and breathing exercises designed to help clients get ready to speak. Klimek, in *Balancing Breath and Tone* (Chapter 4), leads the client through a self-exploration of easy, comfortable breathing. And Lader and Wolf's *Alexander-Based Vocal Therapy* (Chapter 6) provides guidance for a journey in self-awareness of breathing in different body positions.

As you plan your session goals directed toward improving your client's speech-breathing support, we urge you to peruse the other sections of this book. You will find a delightful variety of approaches to breathing interwoven throughout many of the exercises.

Why Don't You?

Alison Behrman

Purposes

To promote:

- Self-awareness of breathing as the energy supply for speech and the process of replenishing and releasing.
- Coordination of breath supply with phrasing demands in conversational speech.
- Vocal expression (pitch, loudness, and rhythm).

Origin

A popular exercise that I have often seen therapists use for improving speech breathing is to have the client count a progressively increasing series of numbers, such as 1 {breath}, 1–2 {breath}, 1–2–3 {breath}, and so forth. Another variation that I have observed is to use a series of sentences of increasing length. Here I combine the two exercises and use progressive-length sentences, with each sentence incorporating the prior phrase and building on it. An actor I worked with had particular fun using different emotions with each repetition. I have since found that many nonactors find this exercise a good opportunity to release their "inner actor" and work on expression (pitch and loudness variation and rhythm) along with breathing.

Overview

This exercise is designed primarily to help the client manage speech-breathing support. However, as the client becomes adept at breath control, the therapist can shift the focus of the exercise to vocal expression, encouraging greater variety of pitch, loudness, and rhythm. By encouraging the client to have fun with the exercise, the mood of the therapy session can become light and energetic, a nice change of pace from the sometimes serious discussions about managing vocal demands and compliance with home practice assignments.

The Exercise

1. Place a copy of the following sentences in front of you at a comfortable height and distance so that you can sit or stand

Optional: Negative practice: After you have achieved some success using good speech-breathing support while reading, go back to the old way of breathing and feel the difference. Try taking in too little or too much breath before the start of the phrase. Try to complete the lengthier phrases on a single breath.

Optional: Expression practice: Practice the phrases using good speech-breathing support while you focus on different aspects of expression, including pitch, loudness, and rhythm. Try making the pitch move up and down more than usual (a little "singsong"). Try speaking the phrases more loudly or more softly while maintaining appropriate speech-breathing support. Or try to vary the loudness level within each phrase, making some words softer than others. And experiment with the rhythm—the internal timing of the phrase—reading some syllables more slowly than others, and inserting slight pauses of varying duration between words. As you vary all of these expressive aspects, make sure to match your changes with the meaning of the words. You could also try to change the expression by reading with different emotions: sad, angry, happy, excited, teasing, provocative, or sarcastic, for example.

easily with your upper torso erect but relaxed, your shoulders even, and your head well-balanced on your neck, facing forward. (Avoid placing the sentences flat on a desk where you have to bend over or tuck your chin downward to read.)

2. Take a relaxed, oral breath and read the first phrase. Allow the excess air to be released at the end of the phrase. Repeat the relaxed breath for each subsequent phrase. Avoid taking in so much air that you build up a sensation of tension in your upper torso (overbreathing). For the lengthier phrases, you will probably be most comfortable if you take a second, smaller breath part of the way through the reading.

"Why?"

"Why don't you?"

"Why don't you come along?"

"Why don't you come along and help me?"

"Why don't you come along and help me with the shopping?"

"Why don't you come along and help me with the shopping at the grocery store?"

"Why don't you come along and help me with the shopping at the grocery store this morning?"

"Why don't you come along and help me with the shopping at the grocery store this morning before John and Alison come over?"

"Why don't you come along and help me with the shopping at the grocery store this morning before John and Alison come over, and then we can all have lunch?"

"Why don't you come along and help me with the shopping at the grocery store this morning before John and Alison come over, and then we can all have lunch and talk about our plans for the weekend?"

"Why don't you come along and help me with the shopping at the grocery store this morning before John and Alison come over, and then we can all have lunch and talk about our plans for the weekend? It'll be so much fun!"

Breath Pacing

Linda M. Carroll

Purpose

■ To facilitate use of good speech-breathing support, especially breath-pacing, and use of a relaxed catch-breath (a term used by singers for a quick breath in the middle of a phrase).

Origin

I learned this exercise from Bonnie Raphael, a distinguished theatre arts voice trainer.

Overview

This exercise is particularly useful for individuals who rush their breath intake, or who are poor at breath pacing. The client establishes a rhythmic counting and breathing process, with gradually less time for the breath. Rhythmic finger-tapping may be used for each beat of inhalation to establish comfortable pacing. The breath inhalation should encompass the entire breathing time available, and all or most of the breath should be used, down to resting expiratory level, when the counting resumes.

The Exercise

Count out loud from one to 10 at a steady, moderate pace. Then allow four beats for a slow breath intake. (See the pattern diagrammed below. Each asterisk represents one beat for the inhalation breath.) Repeat the counting, allowing three beats for the breath. Continue, reducing the amount of time you allow for the breath, until you have to "catch" a breath without a beat.

"1-2-3-4-5-6-7-8-9-10"-*-*-*-*

"1-2-3-4-5-6-7-8-9-10"-*-*-*-*

"1-2-3-4-5-6-7-8-9-10"-*-*-*

"1-2-3-4-5-6-7-8-9-10"-*-*-*

"1-2-3-4-5-6-7-8-9-10"-*-*

The late Carol N. Wilder, Ph.D., professor of speech-language pathology at Columbia University, taught a similar exercise to train quick inhalation. The client and therapist count and clap four sets of 8 at a medium rate, with a quick, quiet breath between each set. If the client can manage the quiet inhalation with no easing of the clapping rhythm, then sets of 9 and 10 may be attempted.

"1-2-3-4-5-6-7-8-9-10"*-*

"1-2-3-4-5-6-7-8-9-10"*

"1-2-3-4-5-6-7-8-9-10"*

"1-2-3-4-5-6-7-8-9-10" (catch breath)

"1-2-3-4-5-6-7-8-9-10" (catch breath)

"1-2-3-4-5-6-7-8-9-10"

"1-2-3-4-5-6-7-8-9-10"

Clients who have difficulty with breath management from "1-2-3-4-5-6-7-8-9-10" can shorten the exercise to "1-2-3-4-5-6-7" until sufficient breath pacing during phonation is established.

Breathing Awareness

Ellen Love Dungan and John Haskell

Purposes

- To increase the client's awareness of breathing during speech, specifically, the breath as energy and the process of replenishing and releasing.
- To help coordinate breath supply with phrasing demands in conversational speech.

Origin

These exercises were developed for voice workshops that we conducted for a number of years at Columbia University. Many of the students in the groups had poor speech–breathing habits, such as excessively long breath groups, gasping for breath, and mistiming of voice onset. One of the goals for the students was to integrate new breathing skills into their conversational speech, and, in order to accomplish this, they had to start monitoring their breathing during speech. They had to learn that they could make decisions about when to take breaths and how much air to inhale. (Later, in using these exercises with actors, we learned that "Creative Counting" is similar to exercises used in some acting classes, though probably with a different purpose.)

Overview

The therapist should introduce the exercises with the idea that, although breathing is an automatic function, one can make choices about the breathing process. One can breathe because one needs to, or because one chooses to shape an utterance in a particular way. In these exercises, the client moves from counting, with designated breathing, through a sequence of exercises toward spontaneous speech, with breathing choices made along the way. As expected, the client usually finds that he or she is less aware of the breathing process as the language demands increase. The ultimate goal is a balance between concentration on the ideas to be communicated and general monitoring of breathing. During the exercises, the self-monitoring increases if the client places a hand on his or her lower ribs and stomach area.

The Exercises

1. Counting to 20
   Count to 20 at a comfortable rate, smoothly connecting the numbers. Take a relaxed breath after every five numbers.

2. Creative Counting
   Count to 30 at a comfortable rate. Take breaths as needed and/or desired. (For example, you may feel your air supply getting low, but you may decide to wait a few numbers before inhaling. Or, you may decide to take a pause and a breath before you actually need to.) Be sure to take enough time to inhale quietly.

   Do the exercise again with excitement in your voice. Tell a story about something very exciting, only tell it with numbers, and remember to breathe.

   > *Optional*: Counting in Conversation
   > (The client and therapist count to 40 conversationally, each counting as far as he/she wants, then letting the other continue; then back and forth. Both client and therapist must monitor breathing.)

3. Carrier Phrases
   Look around the room and identify objects, using carrier phrases of increasing length (see below). Be sure to take a comfortable breath for each sentence.

   > I see a _____ and a _____.
   > I see a _____ and a _____ and . . . (etc.).
   >
   > That is a _____ and a _____.
   > That is a _____ and a _____ and . . . (etc.).
   >
   > Where is the _____ and the _____?
   > Where is the _____ and the _____ and . . . (etc.)?

4. Sequence of Events (Daily activities, instructions, directions)
   State six to eight activities that you generally do during the day. Say each activity in a short, simple sentence, taking a breath after the sentence. Keep the activities in sequential order.

   > *Example:* I wake up at 6:30.
   >   I get dressed and eat breakfast.
   >   Then I take the subway to work.
   >   At work I first read the mail.
   >   Then I make some phone calls.
   >   At about 10 o'clock there is usually a meeting.

Repeat the activities using a more natural speaking style. You may combine two or three activities in extended sentences. Remember to breathe as needed or desired.

Example: I get up at 6:30 and get dressed and eat breakfast. (*Breath*)
or
I get up at 6:30 and get dressed. (*Breath*) Then I eat breakfast and leave for work. (*Breath*)

5. Monologue
Talk extemporaneously for about one minute, relating an incident or commenting on an issue or event. Remember to breathe comfortably along the way.

Flow Phonation

Jackie Gartner-Schmidt

Purposes

To facilitate increased:

■ Airflow management in speech.
■ Ease of phonation.
■ Forward oral resonance through focus on balanced airflow.

Origin

This exercise was inspired by the concept of *flow phonation* as introduced by Gauffin and Sundberg (1989) and the therapeutic approach "Stretch and Flow Phonation" (Casteel & Stone, 1997).

Overview

This exercise provides a visible cue to facilitate increased airflow in speech. A facial tissue positioned near the lips is used as biofeedback to help the client achieve increased awareness of airflow energy at the front of the mouth and its connection to voice production. Then, a hierarchy of speech tasks is used to train the use of flow phonation in contrast to **breathy** or **pressed** phonation. This exercise may be helpful particularly with clients who frequently exhibit breath-holding behaviors when speaking.

Note: The therapist demonstrates each step of the exercise before the client performs the task.

The Exercise

1. Take a strip of facial tissue and hold it between your index and third fingers, approximately two inches from your nose. Take a breath and exhale a sigh with a voiceless /u/, as though you had just finished a long, hard day and you are sighing with relief. The tissue should move with the airflow. Repeat until accuracy is achieved consistently.

2. Keep the facial tissue in the same position and produce the following phrases without voicing. Although no voiced sound is

---

The reason a voiceless /u/ is used is because the lip contour for /u/ directs the airflow in a column from the lips and it is easy to move the tissue and hear a steady airflow stream. As the client produces the voiceless /u/, the therapist should pay attention to any hesitation (breath-holding) that may occur at the top of the inhalation just before the exhalation occurs. The cycle of inhalation followed by exhalation on a voiceless /u/ should be produced smoothly and without hesitation. If done properly, the tissue will be uplifted by the airflow and the sound of the airflow will be smooth and steady. Unsteady airflow may be a sign of breath-holding and/or excessive constriction of the vocal tract. On achieving a steady airflow, the client should be asked to comment on the degree of effort used to produce the voiceless /u/. The goal is to achieve the task with minimal effort.

produced, you are moving the articulators around the steady stream of airflow. The tissue should move with the airflow. Within each phrase, connect each of the syllables or words together, so that no separation or pausing occurs. Examples of phrases are:

Poo-loo- poo-loo- poo-loo

Who is Lou?

Who is Sue?

Who are you?

3. Repeat Step 1, but add voicing. Take a breath and exhale on /u/ in a downward glide like a sigh. The tissue should move with the airflow. The sound you produce should be breathy, smooth and steady, and little effort should be felt. Repeat until accuracy is achieved consistently.

4. Contrast breathy and flow phonation styles. First, produce breathy phonation on an /u/ as in Step 3, using the tissue to monitor airflow. Make note of the breathy quality of the sound. Then produce an /u/ again, but this time, produce a non-breathy sound yet achieve the same movement of the tissue. This manner of voice production is called flow phonation.

> Often, the only cuing needed for the client for production of flow phonation is to ask for a less breathy sound, or to increase the loudness of the sound.

5. Contrast pressed and flow phonation styles. First, produce an /u/ again but do not allow any airflow to move the tissue. Now produce /u/ using flow phonation, allowing the tissue to move but without the breathy voice quality. Contrast the sensation and degree of effort for pressed and flow phonation styles.

As the use of the tissue is faded, direct the client to focus on the sensation of energy in the front of the mouth instead of the airflow. The use of voiceless fricatives can be helpful for establishing this sensation of energy, proceeding then to the voiced cognates.

The therapist may elect to preface this exercise by introducing the concepts of breathy, flow, and pressed phonation styles. The continuum below, adapted from Gauffin and Sundberg (1989), can be shown to the client, and the therapist can provide a definition (see Glossary) and phonatory model of each type of phonation.

> Breathy Phonation→
> Flow Phonation→Pressed Phonation

6. Repeat the phrases used in Step 2, but this time use flow phonation. Make sure that the tissue is moving with the airflow but that the sound is not breathy. Alternate productions of breathy, flow, and pressed phonation as necessary to help establish the use of flow phonation.

7. Repeat Steps 2 through 6 without the use of the tissue. Once you are able to produce flow phonation consistently and easily and contrast flow phonation with breathy and pressed phonation, move on to practice words and phrases starting with voiceless and voiced fricatives to encourage airflow (without the use of the tissue). For example:

> See
> See Sally
> See Sally sleep
> See Sally sleep soundly
> See Sally sleep soundly by the sea
>
> Zebras
> Zebras zigzag
> Zebras zigzag at
> Zebras zigzag at the Zoo
>
> Vince
> Vince vowed
> Vince vowed to vote

8. The final key to using flow phonation in conversational speech is to allow articulation to facilitate the sensation of energy at the front of the mouth. Practice using flow phonation while maintaining awareness of articulatory activity first with sentences that include many phonemes produced in the front of the mouth. The following sentences may be helpful.

> Teachers eat ripe peaches at the beach.
>
> Fat Freddy prefers french fries.
>
> You should polish your purple shoes.

When accuracy is achieved consistently, practice flow phonation and articulatory clarity in conversation.

Relaxed Heart-Mind Breathing

Susan Miller

Purposes

- To prepare the mind and body for speaking under stress.
- To reduce speech-related anxiety.

Origin

Stone seals in the Indus Valley dating back to around 3000 BC show Yogic postures and the earliest evidence of Yoga. The art of yoga consists of eight disciplines, one of which, Pranayama, deals with the regulation of breath. Breathing techniques have long been used by yoga teachers, Lamaze teachers, and even anesthetists to elicit a state of relaxation. Professional athletes who need to diminish their physiologic arousal but maintain alertness and energy practice deep breathing and a positive emotional state. It is hypothesized that these techniques can lead to a high performance state. Public speakers often are taught these techniques with the goal of remaining relaxed yet focused and energized.

Overview

This exercise is a modification from a classic yoga exercise, in which air is inhaled deeply through one naris followed by breath holding and exhaling and then inhalation through the other naris, holding, and exhalation. In this exercise air is inhaled through the nose with the tongue in a forward position so that the throat remains open. Air moves into and out of the lower thorax easily. After several breaths the client is asked to imagine that the breath comes into and out of the area around the heart. As the client breathes "into the heart" she or he is asked to think of someone or something that is appreciated. The goal of this exercise is to establish a coherent heart rate rhythm which is hypothesized to energize you and increase your ability to focus keenly. The exercise is based on the assumption that although a person can't always control the events that will occur, a person can learn to control one's emotions to remain relaxed yet focused to reach one's target.

The Exercise

1. Inhale and exhale easily through your nose with your jaw relaxed and your face long (as if you were performing a nasal or "stifled" yawn with your lips closed). Allow air to come naturally into your lower thorax and back out. Try not to hold your breath either at the peak of inhalation or the end of exhalation. You will not move large amounts of air. Follow your breathing as it becomes smoother.

2. Relax your tongue by placing your tongue tip lightly behind your upper front teeth or lightly behind your lower front teeth. This tongue placement will help to open the back of your throat and allow the needed amount of air to come in automatically. You do not need to inhale or suck in large amounts of air, which could result in increased tension.

3. When your breathing is smooth and balanced, pretend that your breath is flowing in and out of your heart. Now find a positive feeling like appreciation for a special person, a pet, a place that you enjoy, or an activity that you enjoy. Close your eyes and breathe "into and out of your heart" as you think of this appreciation. Focus on how much love you feel or how great you felt during or after the event. Visualize it, feel it, and sense it.

Chapter 4

USING A SEMIOCCLUDED VOCAL TRACT

What happens when you produce sound with a narrow opening in the oral cavity, as would occur by lightly placing a hand over the mouth or setting the lips or tongue into rapid vibration? Using the term *semioccluded vocal tract*, Titze (2006) explains that these maneuvers increase the interaction between the airflow directed by the vibrating vocal folds and the resonance features of the vocal tract. Exercises that use a semi-occluded vocal tract engage the voice production system across multiple levels—breathing, phonation, and resonation. Because of the relative occlusion, the sound produced is not very loud and the force with which the vocal folds collide is minimized. Thus, the client may be free to engage fully the breathing system and experience the strong vibratory sensation of forward oral resonance without the inhibition sometimes associated with making loud sounds, and without the concern of phonotrauma. Voice therapists, teachers of theater voice (Lessac, 1960; Linklater, 1976), as well as singing teachers have incorporated the concept of a semioccluded vocal tract into vocal exercises for many years.

Seven exercises are included in this section. Behlau and Madazio's *Combined Flexible Straw Phonation Sequence* introduces the process of phonation with a semioccluded vocal tract, first with the client blowing bubbles through a straw, and then without the bubbles. Behlau and Oliveira's *Hand-Over-Mouth* allows the client to achieve the sensation of forward resonance during speech by placing a hand over the mouth. Extending this sensation of forward resonance is the commonly used lip or tongue trills. Rapid release of the occlusion during phonation helps the client maintain a vocal tract posture that facilitates resonant voice production. Another exercise based on Titze's idea is Rosenberg's *Wave in a Cave*. The cave is formed by the closure of the hands in front of the mouth. Starting with a neutral vowel and changing in pitch, the client progresses through rote speech to higher levels of speech complexity. Four exercises in this chapter, Behrman's *Lip Buzzes*, Gherson's *Trilled Carryover*, Klimek's *Balancing Breath and Tone*, and Petty's

Tongue Bubble Glides, share the approach of vibrating the lips or tongue tip. Identified by many different names—flubs, flutters, bubbles, buzzes, Bronx cheers, raspberries, and trills—these exercises cannot be traced back to a specific origin, but it is likely that actors and singers used them long before they were adopted by voice therapists.

Other means of partially occluding the vocal tract include use of voiced fricatives, such as /v/ and /ð/, or phonating through a straw (Titze, 2006) or glass tube (Laukkunen et al., 1995). Many other exercises in this book capitalize on a semioccluded vocal tract, particularly with the use of nasals, to facilitate a sensation of forward resonance, including particularly Carroll's *NG Sniff*, Haxer's *Hyperfunctional Dysphonia*, Lader's *Chant Talk*, Schneider's *Hum-Sigh with Chewing*, and Yiu's *Hong Kong Humming* (all found in Chapter 5).

Combined Rigid and Flexible Straw Phonation Sequence

Mara Behlau and Glaucya Madazio

Purposes

- To decrease vocal tract constriction and supraglottic involvement
- To reduce the collisional force of the vocal folds
- To produce more efficient voicing.

Origin

The idea of using a tube for phonation in order to improve voice quality has been practiced in Scandinavia since the 19th century (Laukkanen, 1992). Here, we present a combined sequence using a wide, flexible straw in water to introduce and practice the technique, followed by a narrower, rigid straw in air that offers greater resistance to the airflow. We learned the flexible technique directly from our Finnish colleague, Marketta Sihvo, many years ago at the Pacific Voice and Speech Foundation Conference. She called this technique Sihvo Lax Vox Method (Lv) (Sihvo & Denizoglu, 2007). We learned the use of a high-resistance, rigid straw from Ingo Titze (Titze, 2000, 2006).

Overview

The first set of exercises uses a wide diameter, flexible straw with the end inserted into water; the second set uses a shorter, narrow-diameter, rigid straw without water. The sequence of exercises should be practiced at least 3 times a day to facilitate improved glottic closure and ease of vibration. If the goal is to reduce vocal fatigue and improve endurance, we suggest increasing the practice up to 8 times a day. The exercises can also be used as a first step for a vocal warm-up.

The Exercises

Flexible Straw Into the Water

1. Fill a small (250-mL) bottle, such as a soda or water bottle, with room temperature water. Insert a wide, flexible straw, approximately 14 inches long and at least a quarter of an inch in

diameter (35 cm long by 9 mm in diameter), approximately 1 inch (2 to 3 cm) below the water's surface. Use a shorter straw for children.

2. Standing with good posture, and holding the bottle and straw with your hands, put the straw gently between pursed lips, as though you were going to sip through it.

3. Produce a neutral, sustained vowel sound through the straw. Do not try to achieve a specific sound. Your voicing should cause the water to bubble and you should begin to have a sensation of back pressure or reverberation (resonation) in your mouth and throat. If you do not experience this sensation, slowly increase the pressure (loudness). Continue for one minute, inhaling through your nose as needed. Maintain a relaxed vocal tract and avoid puffing out your cheeks with air. If you feel tension or discomfort or your cheeks become distended, reduce the air pressure slightly as you maintain voicing until your cheeks and vocal tract relax. Then, slowly increase the pressure again.

4. Repeat step 3, progressing up to 3 minutes.

5. Once again repeat step 3, this time varying the depth of the straw as you phonate the neutral vowel. Notice that the sensation of resonation in your mouth and throat, and the amount of pressure required to maintain voicing, vary with the depth of the straw in the water.

6. Sing a tune wordlessly, such as "Happy Birthday," while phonating into the straw.

Rigid Narrow Plastic Straw Into the Air

1. For this exercise, use a rigid straw approximately 3.5 inches long and a tenth of an inch in diameter (9 cm long and 2 to 3 mm in diameter). Use a shorter straw for children. Standing with good posture, and holding the straw with one hand, put the straw firmly between pursed lips, as though you were going to sip through it.

2. Produce a neutral, sustained vowel sound through the straw, similar to the first exercise. Continue for one minute, inhaling through your nose as needed. You should have a sensation of back pressure or reverberation (resonation) in your mouth and throat. If you do not experience this sensation, slowly increase the pressure (loudness). Make sure that no air leaks out between your lips around the outside of the straw, or through your nose, and that your cheeks are not bulging outward. If leakage or bulging occurs or you experience tension or discomfort, reduce the air pressure and then slowly increase it again.

3. Repeat step 2, progressing up to 3 minutes.

4. Next, purse your lips and produce a sustained "oo" sound. Try to maintain the same vocal quality and sensations that you had experienced when using the straw. Repeat 3 times.

For both exercises, encourage the client to monitor sensory changes, such as an easier phonation and a clearer vocal quality. Modeling during the exercise is essential to control posture, breathing coordination, and upper resonance focus.

After completion of each exercise sequence, explore voicing without the straw while trying to maintain a sensation of resonance in your mouth and throat. Start first with a voiced yawn; then, move on to words and short sentences that contain many nasal and fricative consonants; finally, progress to poems and longer speech segments.

Hand-Over-Mouth

Mara Behlau and Gisele Oliveira

Purposes

- To reduce vocal tract constriction.
- To produce more efficient voicing.
- To increase frontal/oral resonance.

Origin

This exercise was inspired by our search for alternatives to the yawn-sigh and other open mouth techniques that are used commonly to reduce constriction along the vocal tract. Our goal was to develop a technique that would allow the client to experience an easily obtained and rapid change in voice production. After some exploration, we came up with an almost extreme mouth closure, without involving the nose cavity, followed by a sudden release. We published an earlier version of this exercise in 1994 (Behlau, 1994). A decade later, Titze (2006) addressed the acoustic features of a group of maneuvers that share a feature he identified as a "semi-occluded vocal tract." His exercises included phonating through straws of varying diameter, producing bilabial or labiodental voiced fricatives, lip or tongue trills, nasal consonants, and the vowels /u/ and /i/. Our exercise can be included in that group.

Overview

This exercise uses the closure of the mouth while producing a stable sound to free constrictions along the vocal tract. The client is encouraged to monitor sensations of openness along the vocal tract and vibrations around the lips and in the hand that is over the mouth. On release of the hand, the goal is for the client to maintain the nonconstricted vocal tract during phonation, perceiving a clearer and more easily produced voice.

Note: The client should be instructed to use this exercise several times during the day, particularly during episodes of prolonged talking, in order to habituate the nonconstricted vocal tract posture.

The Exercise

1. Open your mouth and place the palm of one hand over your mouth, so that your mouth is almost but not completely occluded.

2. With the hand still covering the mouth, produce a sustained neutral sound. It will resemble a *buzz*. Do not try to achieve any specific vowel. Do not inflate your cheeks. You should feel some air going through your fingers and vibrations in your hand and around your lips. Repeat from 5 to 10 times and focus on the sensation of an open vocal tract and easy production of sound. If you experience discomfort from the pressure in your vocal tract, reduce the pressure of your hand against your mouth a small amount, or reduce loudness a bit. You may also want to start with only three repetitions, and slowly build up to 10 repetitions.

3. Remove your hand from your mouth and produce an open vowel, such as /ɑ/. Try to achieve the same sensation of an open vocal tract and easy production of sound.

4. Practice with words, phrases, and then sentences, particularly those loaded with nasals or fricatives.

Wave in a Cave

Marci Daniels Rosenberg

Purposes

- To relax the vocal tract musculature
- To facilitate a resonant hum
- To maximize efficient vocal fold vibration.

Origin

This exercise was inspired by the semioccluded vocal tract exercises described by Titze (2006) and the Hand-Over-Mouth exercise by Mara Behlau and Gisele Oliveira in this volume.

Overview

The underlying principle of this exercise is that occlusion at the front of the vocal tract creates a back-pressure that, in turn, allows for vocal fold vibration to occur in a slightly abducted position. This reduces the collisional forces of the vocal folds during phonation (Titze, 2006). The key to success with this exercise is helping the client to experience maximum vibration and "bounce back" of sound with little effort. Allow the client to play with the exercise until he or she discovers the "sweet spot." Cue the client to listen and feel for a hollow, reverberant sound. The shape of the "cave" formed by the hands is important: the closure of the hands should be neither too closed nor too open. This exercise is a helpful starting point for the patient having difficulty achieving relaxed, resonant hum. Once the exercise is performed correctly, the client should notice a re-calibration of the speaking voice that is easier and better placed.

The Exercise

1. Create the cave by cupping both hands together as if around a baseball. The thumbs encircle each other creating the opening.
2. Generate a neutral vowel sound into the opening of the "cave" that you have created with your hands. The throat should feel open and relaxed.

3. Glide up and down in a natural speech-based pitch contour that is similar to a siren. Continue until you are able to produce target sound without cueing or modeling from the therapist.
4. Once the glide is stable, build on this by increasing the pitch contour and by adding rote speech and then more complex speech tasks.
5. Vary the tasks, returning to the basic gesture if needed.

Lip Buzzes

Alison Behrman

Purposes

- To warm up the voice.
- To increase speech-breathing support.
- To increase vocal fold elongation and amplitude of mucosal wave vibration without excessive impact stress.

Origin

Lip buzzes are among the first exercises that I teach to all of my clients. When I first started using lip buzzes, I sensed that many clients who started immediately with a glide were rushing the exercise and focusing mainly on the extent of the upward glide. By starting with the simpler task of a sustained pitch, the client has an opportunity to focus on the process of engaging the breath fully, maintaining a relaxed vocal tract, and sensing the almost effortless production of voice. The **messa di voce** maneuver included in this exercise was inspired from a presentation at a Pacific Voice Conference by Rosemary Ostrowski.

Overview

This variation of lip buzzes begins with sustained tones at different pitches, followed by progressively widening glides, and then ends with a messa di voce produced at different pitches. This exercise may be particularly appropriate for clients with excessive muscular tension and may be helpful for vocal fold scar.

Note: It can be particularly helpful for the client to sip water to maintain moist lips during this exercise. Guide the client to focus on a sensation of open throat and sound pressure against the inside of the lips, with the target being effortless voice production. Remind the client that the focus is on the *process* and not the sound produced.

The Exercise

1. Select a pitch in your usual speaking range and sustain the tone with the buzz. Put a fair amount of voice behind the lips (in other words, don't make it all lip buzz without voiced sound). Focus on the sensation of vibration at the lips and an open throat.

Some clients may need to touch gently the sides of the cheeks close to the lips with one finger on each side of the mouth to assist in achieving the buzz. If the lips stop or the buzz cannot be maintained adequately, encourage your client by saying that difficulty with the task is normal. Explain that it just means that there is a bit too much tension in the lips and an uneven breath support. Help the client to focus on a steady breath pressure driven from control of the abdominal muscles, not the throat.

2. Repeat at three progressively higher pitches. The notes you select are not critical to the success of the exercise.
3. Slide from a low to a high pitch. Repeat this slide four or five times. With each repetition, widen the slide just a bit (starting a bit lower and going a bit higher). Do this task slowly.
4. Return to the pitch at which you began this exercise in Step 1. This time, perform a messa di voce at a single pitch. That is, start softly and build to a moderately louder sound and then slowly fade to a softer sound. Perform one soft-loud-soft manuever per breath. Allow the same amount of time (generally about two beats) for each part of the soft-loud-soft task. Do not fade rapidly at the end but instead maintain control through the end of the task.
5. Repeat the messa di voce at three progressively higher pitches.

Balancing Breath and Tone Through Advanced Trill/Flutter Tasks

Mary McDonald Klimek

Purposes

- To facilitate improved speech-breathing support and balance of airflow with laryngeal muscle activity.
- To warm up the voice.
- To cool down the voice.

Origin

Many voice teachers and voice therapists employ trill/flutter tasks as breathing and tone production exercises. My experiences with lip trills go back to when I was a singing student. I was running out of breath on a phrase, and my teacher, Robert Gartside, had me lip trill through the phrase. I remember being struck by the sensation of using more breath to trill than I had while singing and being surprised when I actually made it all the way through (on my second attempt). When I sang the phrase using the same "gesture of breath" (a term I use which may have originated with Bob Gartside), I made it through with breath to spare! Later, as a graduate student at the Voice and Speech Laboratory at Massachusetts Eye and Ear Infirmary in Boston, I observed Patricia Benjamin Doyle demonstrating a masterful array of lip trill tricks, turning her voice off and on and changing pitches without a single bobble or hesitation in her lip flutter.

Overview

These exercises use flutters and trills to achieve balance of the voice production system and to explore the client's "inner rules." Inner rules are assumptions made by the client about how the voice production system *works* under different conditions (of pitch and loudness, for example). Inner rules guide the speaker in routine conversation as well as within special vocal demands such as performance, public speaking, or telephone conversations. For singers, exploration of the inner rules that guide their speaking voices sets the stage for revising breath-tone connections in their singing voice. Some of the inner rules of breath-tone management discussed here play a part in the deterioration of performing voices.

The exercises described here are informative to a wide range of voice clients. The exercises take only a few minutes to address within a therapy session. Typically, I work hierarchically and let the client settle into successful demonstration of one task before introducing the next. I often model with my fingers or hands, miming the plane and movement of the true vocal folds. One can trill into various nasal hums (the basic training gestures of resonant voice therapy). Well-produced trills can set the stage for vocal recovery by restoring overall vocal balance, with the trills becoming key components of vocal warm-up and cool-down routines later during the maintenance stage of therapy.

Note: It is assumed that the client:

- has been introduced to the basic biomechanics of voice production.
- has performed relaxation exercises and stretches.
- is able to maintain a comfortably upright posture, well balanced, and with appropriate spinal curvature.
- is capable of quiet breathing with gentle and appropriate inward and outward movement centered in the middle of the torso (low thoracic, abdominal).

The Exercises

I. Monitoring for Sufficient and Steady Flow of Breath

In this first task, voiceless flutters are used to train "just right breath" (neither too much nor too little) supplied evenly to the glottis throughout a comfortable range of lung volumes, relying on elastic recoil forces rather than active abdominal contraction for exhalation.

1. Find and experience resting expiratory level (REL), the place where the body reaches a resting "balance point" at the end of a natural exhalation. REL is found by inhaling and letting the breath go in a silent "whew!"
2. Prepare for the trill/flutter with a "comfortable breath" or *easy* inhalation comfortably above REL. Continue in the breathing cycle and exhale only so far as REL, avoiding the use of abdominal squeezing to move into expiratory reserve. Note that sometimes it can be useful to pause momentarily at REL, waiting for the natural physiologic impulse to inhale in order to discover a "comfortable breath."
3. Choose the voiceless trill/flutter task that comes most easily (facial massage may help the recalcitrant lip trill). Try voiceless lip trills, tongue trills, "raspberries."
4. Perform three voiceless flutter/trills in succession, all on comfortable breaths. Note that this exercise is not a contest of duration.

The goal is to maintain an even trill. Keep the intensity of the trill/flutter constant through the exhalation. If in doubt about where REL lies, simply discontinue the trill/flutter sooner than later and exhale easily until REL is found.

> The trill functions like a "meter" to monitor rate of breath flow. Make sure the breath flow does not "surge" at the start or "fade" at the end.

5. Once an even trill is achieved, consider the sensation of breath flow through the trill. With hands placed at either side of the rib cage at or above the waist in the center of the abdomen, consider the sensation of breath flow as reflected by the inward movement of the abdominal wall and rib cage. Notice the sensations of effort in the mouth and in the torso. (There is no right or wrong here, just observation. However, you may be surprised to find the experience of effort in the torso is less than that in the mouth.)

II. Voicing on Steady and Sufficient Flow of Breath

In this second task, the challenge is to add voicing to the even trill of Task I. The goal is to avoid exceeding the bounds of a comfortable breath, all the while maintaining exactly the same feeling as in the voiceless trill. The internal kinesthetic sensation should be similar to the voiceless trill. Tactile monitoring in the center of the abdomen at or around the waist line should also provide a similar sensation of steadiness of breath flow rate during voicing and voiceless trill/flutter. Make sure not to "growl" the trill—that is, avoid use of a pharyngeal/laryngeal tonal focus and maintain a forward (anterior/oral) placement.

1. At the top of a comfortable inhalation and without hesitation, voice the trill from Task I.
2. Establish or enhance the sensation of a forward tonal focus. Try to feel as though the voice originates at the site of the trill, somewhere in the front half of the mouth. Sometimes a pitch glide starting from a slightly higher pitch will help you to achieve this sensation. Alternatively, pretend that you are about to laugh (with or without an actual smile). This "laugh posture" may help achieve a forward focus. For negative practice, try producing a few trills with a growl or pharyngeal tone focus.
3. Now produce the trill/flutter using speaking range pitch glides while maintaining forward focus and an even flow of breath. Glide downward in the trill, as in a statement. Then glide upward in the trill, as if forming a question. And finally, glide up and down in a siren or "cable car" movement.

Common Problems: Investigating the Inner Rules of Voice Production

Did the trills remain even? Uneven trills sometimes result from "inner rules" about breath and pitch, such as:

Inner Rule #1: "I need more breath as the pitch rises."

Inner Rule #2: "I need less breath as pitch falls."

Although these rules appear to be saying the same thing, they actually manifest quite differently. The corrective intervention that restores an even trill will also feel different from one to the other. Have the client practice within the pitch range where the even flutter can be maintained.

III. A Trip to the Laboratory of Vocal Mechanics

This task is actually a series of steps that explores control of the glottis independent of a steady gesture of breath. The goal of each step is to sustain the even trill of Task I while the voice is being turned off and on. Once again, inner rules may be revealed that carry over into speech. Control your pitch while performing these steps, and make sure to remain within the bounds of a comfortable speaking range.

1. Start with a voiceless trill and then begin voicing while continuing to trill.
2. Start a voiced trill and then stop voicing while continuing to trill.
3. Start a voiceless trill and then start and stop voicing repeatedly while maintaining the trill.
4. Extend the number of repetitions of starting and stopping voice production during the sustained trill within the limitations of a comfortable breath. Vary the pitch of each voiced segment.

More Common Problems: Investigating More Inner Rules of Voice Production

It is not unusual to have any number of interesting things go "wrong" as you move though these exercises. Most problems are associated with the client's inner rules of voice production. Let us take a closer look at some of these rules.

Inner Rule #3: "My voice stops when breath stops."

One easy solution is to introduce the client to voluntary glottal opening and closing. This is readily done in the following sequence of instructions:

1. Say "uh-oh."
2. Repeat the "uh-oh" *silently*. (If the client whispers, have him or her exhale down to REL and try the task again with no movement of breath.)
3. Form several silent "uh-ohs" in a row and listen to the small wet "click-y" sounds as you open the glottis. (Give the client time to discover the subtle sounds and sensations associated with these movements.)
4. Hold the glottis open and notice you can breathe; hold the glottis closed and notice that you cannot breathe; now open the glottis and breathe normally.
5. Now that you know you can open and close the glottis, go ahead and repeat Steps 1 through 4 above and see if they are easier.

In some cases, working from a breath locus of control is effective. Performing Task 2 with an intentional increase in the amplitude of the voiceless portion of the trill and/or large arm gesture. Reinforcing the continuity of the "gesture of breath" beyond the voiced segment may break the pattern.

Inner Rule #4: "In order to turn my voice on, I need to press my vocal folds together."

Here is an instructional scenario for reworking this "inner rule":

1. Remember, the moving airstream draws the folds into vibration when they approximate or get near enough to one another that they get entrained.
2. Try to move the folds into the airstream of the trill very slowly and very gently *just* to the point where a very soft voice is heard. *Sneak* the folds in and out of the breath stream. Is the trill even now? If not, make the trill stronger and the tone even softer!
3. Once your trill is even, try letting slightly more of the folds get entrained into vibration, producing a medium-loud tone. The trill should still be even.
4. Try letting *more* of the folds become entrained into vibration, producing a loud tone. The trill should still be even!

Inner Rule #5: "I need more breath to be loud and less breath to be soft."

More breath is not needed. Instead, a longer closed phase of vibration will increase the loudness.

5. Extend the number of repetitions within the limitations of a "comfortable breath" and vary the intensity or volume of each voiced segment. Keep the trill steady as you go!

Trilled Carryover

Shirley Gherson

Purposes

- To facilitate continuous breath support in speech
- To reduce hyperfunction at the level of words and phrases.

Origin

Historically, speech pathologists and voice teachers have used lip and tongue trills to rebalance breath flow during speech and singing. This exercise was inspired by observing Michelle Horman (see her contribution in this volume) transition from a series of sustained trills into speech tasks. By trilling directly into words and phrases, patients would get a clear sense of carryover and application. I began using the *br*-heavy phrases more regularly with patients who had difficulty maintaining consistent breath support through to the end of the phrase.

Overview

This exercise uses the lip and tongue trills at the beginning of a word, which is then carried into a phrase. This carryover helps to initiate an appropriate breath-voice balance that is extended into speech. It is particularly helpful for clients who demonstrate breath-holding when speaking.

The Exercise

1. Begin to lip or tongue trill at a comfortable, conversational speaking pitch. Repeat until the trill is comfortably produced with a steady flow of breath (for more on how to produce lip and tongue trills, see Behrman's Lip Buzzes or Klimek's Trill/Flutter Tasks in this volume).
2. Produce a series of "br" initial words by replacing the "br" with a trill instead. Try to choose words that end in fricatives or voiced consonants to facilitate the sensation of continuous breath flow. You may need to adjust the trill by pushing your cheeks up for extra support during the initial stages of learning. Elongate the trill and the remaining word as well. Draw

your attention to both the preparatory breath required for initiation, and the energy used during the production of the word itself.

Example: Brrrrrrrrrrrrush for the tongue trill (or alternatively, Bbbbbbbbrush for the lip trill)

    a. Brave
    b. Brazen
    c. Broom
    d. Breath
    e. Brine
    f. Brash

3. Use the starter-phrase "Bring me a " to move on to phrases. Use the trill for both *br*-initial words.

    For example:

    a. Bring me a broom
    b. Bring me a brush
    c. Bring me some breath
    d. Bring me a brownie
    e. Bring me some breakfast

4. Phase out the trill with normally produced words and phrases, continuing to pay attention to the sensation of breath flow at the start of words and the continuance of the flow throughout the phrase.

Tongue Bubble Glides

Brian Petty

Purposes

- ■ To relax the jaw and base of tongue.
- ■ To facilitate good speech-breathing support.

Origin

Variations of this exercise are used widely among voice therapists. This version is based on recommendations of my colleague, Mary Sandage. We use it for a wide range of voice clients, including professional singers.

Overview

The exercise uses a forward combination of tongue and lip trill on an upward and downward pitch glide.

Once the client is able to do the exercise easily, the tongue bubble can be started immediately with voicing (omitting the voiceless tongue bubble). If the client has difficulty performing this exercise due to significant muscle tension, ask the client to protrude the tongue farther than he or she thinks it should be protruded. The client may also benefit from using a mirror to ensure that the tongue protrusion is consistent with the therapist's model. Clients who continue to have difficulty with this exercise may produce a lip trill ("motorboat noise") instead. The tongue trill (such as the Italian "r") is generally not a good alternative because anecdotal evidence seems to suggest that it produces more muscular tension than it corrects.

The Exercise

1. Moisten your lips and allow your tongue to lay over your lower lip in a relaxed manner. Close your lips lightly over your tongue, and blow air over your tongue through your closed lips, making the tongue tip and lips vibrate.
2. While vibrating your lips and tongue tip, glide from lowest to highest comfortable pitch (falsetto or highest range) and back down. Take a breath and repeat.

Chapter 5

RESONANT VOICE

All voices resonate to some degree as the sound wave travels from the vocal folds upward through the vocal tract. But as voice therapists, we know that the ways in which we position our vocal tract and articulators can help or hinder the acoustic properties of the voice. Typically, we associate positive characteristics with a "forward" resonance, including maximizing energy, pleasing sound quality, and ease of production. In contrast, we tend to associate negative characteristics with a "back" or "pharyngeal" resonance, including less efficiency and greater effort of voice production, and perhaps a lesser vocal quality.

Often, resonance is an abstract concept for voice therapy clients, making it difficult to translate concept into motor activity such as tongue position or jaw height. Some of the changes in vocal tract postures that we target, particularly modifications to the oropharynx and supraglottis, are out of sight and difficult to sense without considerable practice. And hearing the differences in resonance qualities can be tricky for both client and therapist. As a result, many therapists have found it easier for clients to focus on a physical sensation, such as a buzz or vibration that can accompany a resonance target, rather than focusing on how the voice *sounds*. Alternatively, or in addition to physical sensation, imagery is used to achieve a desired vocal tract posture, such as instructing the client to try to "smile in the back of the throat" or shaping the throat into an "inverted megaphone."

Nine exercises are included in this section. In Carroll's *NG Sniff*, the nasal sound is used in a glissando to help the client target a forward resonance before opening to a vowel sound across different pitches. Haxer's *Hyperfunctional Dysphonia* employs a hum transitioning into using nasals and glides. In Lader's *Chant Talk*, the resonant trigger "mini" facilitates forward resonance during chanting. Phyland's exercise, *Good Vibrations*, is a fun exercise using spoken text from a popular song to help the client find forward resonance. Pinho's *Spaghetti* uses a sipping maneuver to lower the larynx and help achieve improved resonance. Schneider uses a variety of sounds produced in the front of the mouth in *Chant to Speak* to facilitate a resonant chant, whereas her exercise *Hum-Sigh with Chewing*, supplements nasal phrases with chewing movements to achieve a forward resonance. In Morsomme's *How to Improve Vocal Resonance*, the client is positioned with forehead against a wall, which enhances sound vibrations in various areas of the skull. And finally, Yiu's *Hong Kong Humming* incorporates changes in loudness as the resonance target is achieved. Although these nine exercises are featured in this section, the focus on appropriate resonance is a pervasive theme across most of the exercises in the book. We encourage you to explore the resonance features of these and other exercises included in this book as you plan your therapy sessions.

NG Sniff

Linda M. Carroll

Purpose

- To increase the client's awareness of the contribution of resonance in voice production.

Origin

This exercise is part of the training exercise from Directed Energy Vocal Technique (Carroll, 2000), which applies principles of singing techniques in the treatment of dysphonia.

Overview

Clients with voice disorders often focus excessively on the laryngeal contribution to sound production, and not enough on the role of resonance. I believe that all laryngeal pathology is helped by resonance voice exercises. The present exercise, which attempts to balance the control of the sound source (the vibrating vocal folds) with the vocal tract filter function, makes use of a gentle **messa di voce**. The rationale for the diminuendo before ascending pitch change is that softer phonations should allow easier, safer access to higher pitches. The NG-Sniff should be limited to the modal register range for most clients.

The Exercise

1. Produce an ascending **glissando** slide on /ŋ/ or /n/. Feel the sensation of resistance in the oral and nasal cavities. Do not increase your airflow as you increase pitch. The ascending glide should feel like a slow sniff with your mouth open.
2. At the top of the ascending glissando, switch from the /ŋ/ or /n/ to a clear /i/ or /o/ before descending. A moderate **diminuendo** should be accomplished on the lower tone and completed before the change in pitch. The /i/ and /o/ should not be static with regard to loudness level. Slight loud-soft changes should be made while the vowels are sustained.
3. Continue up and down the scale in semitones within the midrange.

Hong Kong Humming

Edwin Yiu

Purposes

To promote:

- Ease of phonation.
- Increased loudness without effort.
- Use of appropriate speaking pitch.

Origin

This exercise was introduced to Hong Kong in the 1960s by the first speech pathologist in Hong Kong, Ms. Cecilia Chan, who was trained in England. Since that time, it has become one of the most popular techniques for addressing voice problems in Hong Kong. This version of the exercise is inspired by the humming techniques as described by Boone and McFarlane (1999) and Harris, Harris, Rubin, and Howard (1998), as well as the Lessac-Madsen Resonant Voice Therapy (LMRVT) described by Verdolini (1999) and resonant voice therapy by Moncur and Brackett (1974).

Overview

This humming exercise targets ease of phonation and appropriate speaking pitch by emphasizing the sensation of resonance (energy) in the oral-nasal region with minimal effort and tension at the laryngeal and neck regions. The exercise uses different types of speech materials that vary in length and context.

Note: The clinician should produce the hum first for the client to use as a model. The exercise is designed to be conducted over eight to 10 weekly sessions with home practice prescribed accordingly. A home practice plan of three times each day is recommended.

The Exercise

The therapist may direct the client to produce the hum for a specific duration, perhaps for a count of three to five. Alternatively, the client could be directed to hold the hum until a consistent oral-nasal buzz is perceived.

1. Produce a hum on a slight upward glide, as though you were responding to someone by asking for clarification (mmm?). Make sure to use an easy onset (not hard glottal attack) to initiate the hum. The jaw should be low and relaxed throughout the hum. Prolong the hum and focus on a sense of vibration along the bridge of the nose and at the lips (an "oral-nasal

buzz"). Note continuous (uninterrupted) airflow during the hum and a sense of easy vibration. Repeat five times, or until accurate production is achieved consistently.

2. Produce the hum and open into a vowel, such as:

mmm /ɑ/

mmm /i/

mmm /u/

Note that the hum leads directly and smoothly into the vowel, without interruption of airflow. Maintain a low, relaxed jaw throughout the vowel. Repeat until an easy, oral-nasal buzz (resonance) is achieved consistently at an appropriate pitch.

3. The hum is now produced and blended smoothly into a hierarchy of progressively more complex utterances. At each level, the hum and utterances should be repeated until an easy, oral-nasal buzz is achieved consistently at an appropriate pitch.

The following hierarchy is suggested, progressing from stimuli that are the most to the least facilitative of oral-nasal resonance.

> The therapist will need to adapt the hierarchy of stimuli for each client. Some clients may find it easier to maintain oral-nasal resonance in short phrases that are loaded with nasal and continuant phonemes, whereas other clients may find it easier to produce monosyllabic words containing a wide variety of initial phonemes.

Sounds:
Vowels
Nasals (/m/ and then /n/)
Continuants
    Glides (/w/, /j/)
    Liquids (/r/, /l/)
Fricatives
Stops

Structure:
Monosyllabic words
Multisyllabic words
Short daily phrases, for example
    How are you?
    I am fine.
    Let's go for a walk.

4. Practice loudness control with oral-nasal resonance. Produce the hum and blend into short daily phrases. Repeat three times, each time using a successively louder voice but maintaining the easy, oral-nasal resonance and appropriate pitch. For example:

mmm how are you?

mmm how are you?

mmm how are you?

> The client should be encouraged to monitor key features during home practice by asking the following questions:
>
> Is the pitch appropriate?
>
> Is the onset of the hum gentle and smooth?
>
> Is good speech-breathing support being used?
>
> Is the hum sufficiently long to achieve the sensation of oral-nasal buzz?
>
> Is the sensation of ease and low effort maintained?
>
> Is the airflow continuous, without interruptions?

5. Fade the use of the hum while maintaining the easy, oral-nasal resonance.

6. Use the hum in a reading passage. Produce the hum at each point marked by double forward slashes (//). For example:

   //One day, //the wind and the sun had a debate //on who was more capable. //While they were talking, //a man dressed in a thick black coat came along. //So they decided to see who was able//to undress the man//with the black thick coat. //The wind started first by blowing very hard. //But, the harder she blew, //the tighter the man held on to his coat. //So the wind gave up eventually. //A while later, //the sun came out//and it became hot. //The man quickly took off his coat. //So//the wind had to admit //that the sun was more capable. (*Fable attributed to Aesop*)

7. Repeat the reading passage without the hum, but maintain the sensation of easy, oral-nasal resonance and appropriate pitch.

8. Prepare a short monologue and practice it maintaining the easy, oral-nasal resonance. If necessary, use the hum to recapture the resonance and appropriate pitch.

9. Practice the forward resonance in conversation, reintroducing the hum as necessary.

Hum-Sigh with Chewing

Sarah L. Schneider

Purposes

- To minimize tension of the tongue and jaw during phonation.
- To elicit increased oral resonance through wider oral-pharyngeal space.

Origin

Chewing is an exercise that I often use and have observed colleagues using to decrease jaw tension and promote increased jaw excursion. (See Haskell's *Chewing Method* [Chapter 7] for more history of this technique.) I learned the hum-sigh to promote resonant voice production from a colleague while working at the Vanderbilt Voice Center. Later, I observed Margaret Baroody, a singing voice specialist, use a hum while chewing as a vocal warm-up for a singer. I combined the two techniques into this exercise for the speaking voice.

Overview

This exercise develops increased frontal oral resonance, signified by a vibration or "buzzy" sensation at the lips, during production of a hum-sigh while chewing. The chewing is then faded when oral resonance is maintained consistently during hum-sigh. This facilitator should be used through a hierarchy of phonatory tasks working to spontaneous speech. Ultimately, the patient is cued to maintain the forward sensation in spontaneous speech without the use of the facilitator.

Note: The therapist should educate the client about the importance of a released jaw and relaxed tongue placement during voice production prior to beginning this exercise.

The Exercise

1. Take an open breath* and release the air into a hum on a sigh or descending glide while chewing. Feel the vibration or 'buzz'

---

*See *Tongue Out Phonation* exercise also by Sarah Schneider (Chapter 7) for explanation of "open breath."

on the lips or around your nose. Repeat several times until the buzz is established.

2. Produce the hum-sigh with chewing again, and now release it gently into repetitions of /m/ plus vowel, such as /mamama/, /mimimi/, and /momomo/. These utterances should then be repeated without chewing, but the sensation of frontal resonance (buzz) and open throat should be maintained throughout the utterance repetition. Remember to begin each trial with an open breath. Repeat until the sensation of frontal resonance is well established.

3. Now use the hum-sigh with chewing as a facilitator of frontal resonance and ease of production into increasingly complex utterances beginning with words, phrases, and sentences, and then progressing to paragraph reading, and finally conversation. Gradually fade the chewing, maintaining the sensation of buzz.

Chant Talk

Joan Lader

Purposes

- To improve vocal placement or tone focus.
- To encourage easy flow phonation and reduce laryngeal tension.
- To reduce hard glottal attacks.

Origin

Chanting is the production of syllables, words, and phrases in legato or linked style on a monopitch. Chanting, and all of its variations, has a long history in voice training, in promoting frontal/oral resonance and good speech-breathing support. This particular version of chanting is derived from singing exercises and resonant voice therapy techniques.

Overview

This exercise elicits forward resonance through chanting. The client is trained to chant using the nonsense word /mini/. The chant is then extended to other words, phrases, and sentences. The chant is faded while the forward resonance is retained in the natural speaking voice.

The Exercise

1. On a comfortable pitch, begin chanting repetitions of /mini/ on a monopitch with both syllables receiving equal stress. Place your fingers across the bridge of your nose in order to feel the resonant "buzz." You may also feel the buzz sensation by sitting in a chair and bending forward with your head hanging down, or by standing in a corner with your face placed close to the wall.
2. Increase the length of chanted /mini/'s (such as /mini/ /mini/ /mini/).
3. Chant the following: /mini/ one {*breath*}, /mini/ eight {*breath*}, /mini/ nine {*breath*}, /mini/ eleven {*breath*}. Make sure to link the word /mini/ with the number that follows it.

> Practice should be done for short periods of time 4 to 5 times a day. Additional practice should include incorporating improved voice in different life situations, such as telephone conversations, speaking over noise (in restaurants or cars, for example), quiet conversation, and stressful situations.

4. When the chant and accompanying buzz sensation feel easy to produce, chant the following: /mini/ one-eight-nine-eleven. Make sure to link all of the words together on a monopitch.

5. Now chant only on /mini/ and speak the numbers one, eight, nine, eleven. Try to maintain a forward resonance when counting. Repeat until the forward resonance is achieved consistently.

6. Speak the numbers again, reducing the initial chant from /mini/ to just /mi/ (followed by one, eight, nine, eleven), and then reducing it again to just /i/, followed by the numbers.

7. Practice chanting a text loaded with voiced consonants, such as the one below. Chant /mi/ before chanting each sentence.

> There is a word of warning that I will give all of you. Always remember, a wounded bear is angry with everyone and will maul you or anyone in range. A bleeding, wounded bear is a mean animal and will go wild when jabbed or bothered in any way. Even a lion will give ground and avoid a wounded or injured grizzly bear. One dumb move and the bear will lunge and grab you, leaving you dead or gravely wounded. In the name of God, beware of the injured or angry bear. Value my warning. Your well-being is on the line. (*Origin unknown*)

8. Now speak the text using the target chant /mi/ before speaking each sentence, trying to achieve the same easy forward focus and flow.

9. Now practice chanting using voiceless consonants with attention to a relaxed jaw during production of the consonant. Chant the following phrase: /mini/ two {*breath*}, /mini/ three {*breath*}, /mini/ four {*breath*}, /mini/ five {*breath*}.

10. String the numbers together by chanting /mini/ two, three, four, five, six {*breath*}, /mini/ seven, eight, nine, ten, eleven.

11. Speak the numbers again, reducing the initial chant to /mi/.

12. Practice chanting text that contains many voiceless consonants, such as the one below.

> I am going to ask that each of you take this warning. Please don't ever forget that an injured bear is mean and will claw you or others nearby. A hurt, bleeding bear is an angry animal who will go wild if poked or teased in any way. Even the lion retreats to get away from a stunned or wounded grizzly bear. A single false move and the bear will charge and paw you, causing death or serious injury. So look out for a wounded or mean bear. Take this advice. It's your safety that's at stake.

13. Speak the text using the target /mi/ before each sentence, trying to achieve the same easy forward focus and flow.

14. Progress to poetry, reading the newspaper, or a magazine employing the same tools.

Chant to Speech

Sarah L. Schneider

Purposes

- To minimize use of glottal fry at the end of an utterance.
- To improve speech-breathing support.
- To elicit increased oral resonance through wider oral-pharyngeal space.

Origin

I observed a similar chanting exercise initially with Shirley Gherson, voice therapist, while working on increased oral-pharyngeal space and increased oral resonance through the ends of phrases in the speaking voice. A variation of this exercise is also described in Sataloff, Baroody, Emerich, and Carroll (2005).

Overview

This exercise is intended to be a chant on sustained pitches. It is not singing. The speechlike chant is developed by sustaining one pitch or a series of pitches that are ascending or descending. Attention should be focused on maintaining increased oral-pharyngeal space, decreased laryngeal tension, and increased oral-resonance throughout the chanted utterance. No glottal fry should be apparent. Once consistency is achieved on the chanted tasks, the client is asked to try to maintain the easy, resonant vocalization, speaking the same utterance without the chant. Tasks should be completed with increasing complexity and ultimately, without the chanted facilitator.

> *Editors' Note:*
>
> Compare the differences between Lader's and Schneider's chanting exercises. Here, Schneider encourages the client to achieve a forward resonance with the chant using a variety of pitches. Lader establishes the chant with a trigger /mini/ and builds more slowly to conversational speech. The different presentations of a similar technique provide a good demonstration of how a basic exercise can be approached in different manners to address the needs of the individual client.

The Exercise

1. With an open breath* and good speech-breathing support, establish consistent chanting on one pitch beginning with words. The chosen pitch should be in the modal speaking range. The pitch may vary from one trial to the next so as not to limit the pitches used. Use of words with initial phonemes that are

---

*See *Tongue Out Phonation* exercise also by Sarah Schneider (Chapter 7) for explanation of "open breath."

If desired, supplement the chanting with the following exercise. Chant on a series of three descending or ascending pitches. For example,

<u>Tell</u>   <u>going?</u>

   <u>me</u>   <u>you</u>

      <u>how.</u>   <u>Are</u>

This task can provide the client with the experience that pitch can change while maintaining the sensation of oral-pharyngeal space and resonance.

articulated at the front of the mouth paired with front vowels (for example, mean, nine, when) may help increase the sensation of frontal oral resonance. Practice chanting on words until oral resonance and ease of phonation together with good speech-breathing support are achieved consistently.

2. Chant on phrases and sentences. Note the consistency of the tone, resonance focus, and ease of production without falling into vocal fry.

3. Now chant a phrase, followed by the same phrase spoken. While alternating from chant to speech, the same ease and quality developed in earlier steps should be maintained while speaking. Complexity of the utterance should be increased gradually as oral resonance and vocal ease are maintained from chant to speech.

4. Gradually fade the chanting, using it only as needed to regain the target resonance.

How to Improve Your Vocal Resonance

Dominique Morsomme

Purposes

- To warm up the voice
- To increase voice placement in the resonators
- To increase proprioceptive control of the voice.

Origin

When I was a flute student in Belgium, I participated in an annual one-week course for student musicians. We practiced our instruments for 6 hours every day. One of our goals was to perfect the quality of our sound, and an advanced student showed us how to better control sound quality by playing with our heads resting against the wall. In this way, we each created a kind of bubble of sound around our heads. Sound reflection against the wall made the resonance of the sound stronger, allowing us to better hear its quality. Accordingly, we would modify our technique, for example, lip tension, in order to improve the sound color and quality.

At one point, as a speech therapist, I remembered this exercise, which I adapted for vocal rehabilitation. With the forehead against the wall, the client can more readily feel the sound vibrations in the face, the cheekbones, the nasal septum, and particularly on the hard palate. This is a good sensory reference for the client who is a good candidate for resonant voice therapy. Control of the voice becomes not just auditory, but also proprioceptive.

Overview

The client rests his or her head against the wall and makes humming sounds at different pitches starting at a medium level. In the next step of the exercise, the client produces glides from a low pitch to a high pitch and vice versa. During the exercise, we ask the client to turn his or her attention to vibratory sensation and how it shifts. This exercise also promotes muscle relaxation of the shoulder girdle. Indeed, part of the body weight is leaning against the wall and the arms dangle alongside the body. This also causes facial muscles to relax and, thus, allows a better placement of the sounds in the upper resonators.

Note: This exercise is very helpful for clients who have difficulty perceiving vocal vibrations in the face, such as those who suffer from chronic sinusitis or whose facial muscles are very tense. If the client has a cold, the sound vibrations transmitted to the face will tend to loosen the mucus that flows through the nose or to the back of the throat. The vibrations experienced can be very relaxing. The real purpose of this exercise is not a specific sound quality, but the impact of vibrations in the face, which, in turn, may facilitate better sound quality. The longer the client practices, the more the vibrations may be felt.

The Exercise

1. Stand in front of a smooth wall at a distance of about 18 inches. (The exact distance is determined by the height and weight of the individual.) Place your forehead, at the hairline, on the wall. The position should be comfortable. Your arms should be able to swing freely alongside your body.
2. Place your tongue on the hard palate, and start humming with an "n" sound. Slide the sound up and down from very low to very high frequencies.
3. Repeat the process described in step 2 above with the back of your tongue on the soft palate. Produce an "ng" sound and slide from a low to a high pitch. The vibration reinforced by the position of the head on the wall should increase the sensation of vibratory fullness in the head.
4. You can vary the exercises any way you like using different sounds and pitches.

Note: For singers, adapt this exercise to include arpeggios or difficult passages of a musical score.

Good Vibrations

Debbie Phyland

Purpose

■ To decrease base of tongue tension and promote sensory awareness of acoustic vibrations in the mouth.

Origin

I was inspired by the 1966 pop song *Good Vibrations* by The Beach Boys. The song is generally well known and provides an excellent linguistic link to the main thrust of my therapy focus—efficient and healthy vocalizations (vibrations). In the original recording, the main chorus "Good, good, good, good vibrations" is sung with a clear voice quality, and what sounds like an exaggerated forward tongue position.

Overview

In this exercise, the client maintains a forward tongue position while speaking the song's refrain, each time within a slightly different task.

The Exercise

1. Start by placing your tongue tip behind your lower front teeth. Maintain that placement throughout the entire sequence and focus on articulating with the body of the tongue high against the palate. Speak the words slowly in a chant (using a single pitch and linking or sliding between words). Make sure to select a comfortable speaking pitch. Prolong the word *vibrations*, particularly the last two syllables. Maintain a forward resonance and clear vocal quality.

   Good, good, good, good vibra:tions

2. After successful practice with the forward resonance chant, repeat the refrain with natural inflection, maintaining the forward tongue position. Prolong the vowel in the third word (good), emphasizing the forward resonance.

   Good, good, goo:ood, good vibrations

> *Optional Singing*
>
> If desired, sing the refrain, maintaining its original musicality.
>
> Good, good, goo:ood, good vibra:tion:s

3. After you are able to use a natural inflection and good forward resonance while speaking the refrain, add a pitch slide up and back (approximately a fifth, for the musically inclined) on the vowel /u/ at the end of the refrain. The goal is to maintain good frontal resonance and clear voice quality.

   Good, good, goo:ood, good vibra:tion:s /u:/

4. Finally, add phrases after the prolonged vowel to practice transfer of the target voice to regular speech.

   Good, good, goo:ood, good vibra:tion:s /u/ *I'm talking with good vibrations*

   Good, good, goo:ood, good vibra:tion:s /u/ *I'm feeling these good vibrations*

   Good, good, goo:ood, good vibra:tion:s /u/ *1, 2, 3,* (and so on).

Spaghetti

Silvia Pinho

Purpose

■ To establish a low laryngeal position during phonation, without tongue compression.

Origin

Yawning has traditionally been used to elongate the vocal tract and reduce hyperfunction of the vocal mechanism. Often, however, when the client intentionally yawns, the tongue is compressed and tenses the larynx. The Spaghetti exercise was inspired by the concept of flow phonation, introduced by Gauffin and Sundberg (1989), in which a low laryngeal position is a prerequisite for balanced muscle tension in phonation.

Overview

The Spaghetti exercise is a good warm-up procedure for elongating the vocal tract before a professional singing or speaking engagement, similar to warming up musculature for physical activity. The exercise involves a slow sipping movement during inhalation. When performing the exercise, the client should keep the jaw relaxed and the lips rounded, as in the /u/ vowel. The dorsum of the tongue should be slightly retracted and elevated. Low (abdominal) breathing should be used. Sipping water when doing the exercise may be helpful to counter the drying effect of the prolonged inhalation.

The Exercise

1. Sip in air slowly as though you are sipping a strand of spaghetti. Keep sipping until the end of the inspiration, while checking for the lowering of your larynx with your fingers. Repeat this step five times, or until you are sure your larynx is lowering in the process.
2. Sip in as before, and say "Ho-Ho-Ho" with a "Santa Claus" voice. Avoid straining or going down to the bottom of your pitch range as you use this voice. Check to make sure your larynx is still in a lowered position. Repeat several times.

3. Sip in as before, and now with a voice of an "English lord," say "Charles! Bring my car!" Vary your pitch up and down as you say this, and, again, check for the lowered position of your larynx. Repeat several times.

Hyperfunctional Dysphonia

Marc Haxer

Purpose

■ To facilitate improved coordination of breathing and phonation in clients with hyperfunctional dysphonias.

Origin

I was introduced to this protocol a number of years ago by my friend and colleague, Jan Lewin, Ph.D. It was her modifications of a protocol that she presented some years earlier on functional dysphonias given by another friend and colleague, Robert E. ("Ed") Stone, Ph.D.

Overview

This exercise addresses hyperfunctional dysphonia that may be present in the absence of observable laryngeal pathology. It begins with a trigger—a voiced sigh. The voicing produced with the trigger is then shaped into balanced voice production.

Note: Before this exercise is begun, the therapist should explain to the client the nature of his or her voice problem, with particular emphasis on the presence of a *normal-appearing* larynx. No time frame is set for working through the tasks. Building and maintaining confidence is crucial to successful outcome.

Note: Steps that are preceded by an asterisk (*) can be performed simultaneously by the therapist and the client, should that be helpful in certain cases. However, the therapist should gradually stop accompanying the client.

The Exercise

1. Relax your shoulders, using a mirror for visual feedback.
2. Establish low (abdominal) breathing, using a volitional outward movement of the abdomen during inhalation and an inward movement during exhalation ("push out/pull in"). Maintain an open mouth and relaxed throat, focusing on a relaxed exhalation with no sound.
3. *Add a breathy sigh on /ɑ/, increasing the duration of the exhalation.

4. *Extend the sigh longer and make it louder.
5. *Transition the sigh to a hum.
6. *Slowly alternate between the closed (very resonant) hum and the open and relaxed sigh, as in /mːɑːmːɑː/ ("mmaammaa") in a chant (monotonic). Another sound combination you might try is /iːjɑːjɑː/ ("eeyahyah").
7. *Produce the hum and smoothly transition into rote speech tasks in a monotonic chant (legato- or linking-style of speech on a single pitch), such as

   "mmmmmone-two-three-four-five"

   "mmmmMonday-Tuesday-Wednesday-Thursday-Friday"

8. *Drop the hum and, instead, use a hand gesture as a visual cue to maintain the chant, increasing the speed as needed to achieve normal rate.
9. Repeat the rote speech tasks maintaining the legato- or linking-style of speaking but, instead of monotone, use a natural pitch contour.
10. Continue with more complex speech material.

Chapter 6

INTEGRATING VOICE PRODUCTION WITH BODY MOVEMENT

Voice is a complex product of the respiratory, phonatory, resonatory, and articulatory subsystems. Yet, voice therapists and teachers of theater and singing voices are well aware of the contribution of the rest of the body to easy, efficient, and beautiful voice production. A portion of the dysfunctional vocal behaviors that many of our clients demonstrate often appears to arise from impaired or limited postural movements.

This section contains five exercises. Horman's *Arm Swing Warm-Up*, derives from Linklater-based theatre voice training methods, utilizing rhythmic arm movements coordinated with vocal exercises. Through body movements, this exercise may help the client engage full breath support and a relaxed vocal tract, facilitating a forward oral resonance. Gherson's *Messa Arm Swing*, inspired by Horman's exercise, incorporates messa-di-voce into the arm swing. Spencer's *Breath Sensitivity Training* uses a multifaceted approach to increase the client's awareness of speech-breathing support and the mind-body connection, drawing on methods from creative expression in acting and Tai Chi. Paseman, in *I Like to Move It, Move It! Kinesthetically Speaking*, has the client coordinate simple stretches and rhythmic body movements with a hierarchy of voicing tasks to release musculoskeletal tension and access full speech-breathing support. Through this exercise, adapted for the typically small space of a voice therapy room, even clients who are not inclined to dance can learn to access a freer voice through body movements. Lader and Wolf's *Alexander-Based Vocal Therapy* draws on Alexander-based theatrical voice technique, in which the therapist guides the client through postural changes to increase the client's kinesthetic self-awareness, free one's breathing, and release hyperfunction in the vocal tract.

When searching for new ideas to energize and free your client's voice, after perusing the Five exercises included in this section, we encourage you to explore many of the other exercises throughout this book. Attention to body position is an excellent preparation for any set of vocalizing drills. And many of the other exercises can be adapted readily to include rhythmic body movements to enhance achievement of a variety of therapeutic goals.

Arm Swing Warm-Up

Michelle Horman

Purposes

To facilitate increased:

- Speech-breathing support.
- Resonance through wider oropharyngeal space.

Origin

This exercise was inspired by my early exposure to theatre voice training methods as practiced by Leigh Smiley (certified Linklater teacher) and Sharon Freed, who had been on the Voice/Speech faculty at The Juilliard School and The Shakespeare Theatre's Academy for Classical Acting. Many of their methods relied on whole body movement to free the voice. I wanted to create a warm-up that freed the body and voice through movement and yet could be utilized in the small physical space in which I saw patients for voice therapy.

Overview

This exercise utilizes a rhythmic swing of the arms in coordination with breathing, lip trills, lip trills blended into words, and phrases. It is important that the therapist model easy, relaxed coordination of movement and phonation throughout the exercise. The primary target of this exercise is to stimulate rib cage expansion and deep breathing through physical action, and to allow the voice production to reflect the continuous and free movement of the arms and breath. Once learned, this exercise can be modified and used as a brief but effective vocal warm-up when time is limited.

Note: The therapist should demonstrate the full exercise before teaching it to the client.

The Exercise

1. Stand with feet hip-width apart, toes facing forward to protect the knees. Swing your arms up over your head, keeping your arms straight, hands open, facing forward, and fingers stretched but not tense. Do not hold the arms up over your head, but rather allow them to swing back down, reaching about 30° behind the body before swinging upward again. Stay upright

throughout the movement. Do not "dive" forward. Allow the natural momentum of the movement to help set the pace of the arm swing.

2. Once a rhythmic repetition of this swing has been established, add a shallow, gentle bounce of the knees as the hands reach the bottom of the swing. (Add one gentle bounce as your arms drop down toward your sides. Add a second gentle bounce as the arms begin to travel back up toward the head. The purpose of these gentle bounces is to keep the knees and hip joints loose.)

3. Now coordinate breathing with the arm swing. Exhale through gently pursed lips as the arms swing downward and back up toward the ceiling. Then inhale through a relaxed mouth during the next arm-swing cycle. Continue this coordinated rhythm for eight breath cycles or until the task is learned.

4. Add phonation. Begin with a descending glide on a lip trill. The trill should begin as the arms swing downward. Repeat four times. Progress to a "siren" glide on a lip trill, starting in the lower range, gliding up as high as is comfortable and back down again. Repeat four times.

5. Now begin with the lip trill and blend directly into a word. Choose words that begin with /br/ and substitute the trill for the /b/. Utilize words that have *open vowels* to facilitate a relaxed jaw. Produce one word on the downswing and one word on the upswing during the same exhalation. For example:

"BBBBrown Eyes" (Replenish breath on next swing.)

Bouncing too deeply can fatigue the thighs. If the client cannot achieve the knee bounces described in Step 2 in a gentle and comfortable manner, eliminate the bounces and advise the client to keep the knees straight but unlocked, or reduce the number of bounces from two to one.

Note that while the therapist and client are simultaneously swinging their arms, the therapist will produce the model while the client is inhaling, and then the client will imitate the therapist's model on the next swing (while the therapist replenishes her breath to be ready to produce the next model). This pattern allows the therapist to choose stimulus sounds, words, and phrases according to the client's immediate needs and frees the client from having to concentrate on a memorized sequence while performing the exercises. Much of the exercise's value lies in its liberating effect.

"BBBBrainy Child"

"BBBBroadly Drawn"

"BBBBriney Wine"

Remember to focus on releasing the airflow for the vowel sound with the swing of the arms.

> Some clients have difficulty producing lip trills. Alternatives to the lip trills include tongue trills and voiceless fricatives. If tongue trills are used, the spoken phrases should begin with trilled /r/'s or /r/ clusters such as /pr/. If voiceless fricatives are used, the phrases should begin with those fricatives.

6. Proceed to other phrases that facilitate resonant voice through increased oropharyngeal space, such as the two examples provided below, repeating the phrase through multiple arm-swings until a replenishing breath is needed. For example:

    Around and around and around and around . . .

    My oh my oh my oh my . . .

    Allow stressed vowels to be lengthened to coordinate with the length of an upward or downward swing.

7. Repeat Steps 5 and 6 while fading out the arm-swings. Fading can be achieved by using progressively smaller arcs. Focus on recreating the sensations of freedom and release of the voice that was achieved through the body movement.

Messa-Di-Voce Arm Swings

Shirley Gherson

Purposes

- To train dynamics of breath support with visual/tactile feedback
- To coordinate loud voice use with adequate breath support
- To reduce musculoskeletal tension associated with loud voice.

Origin

This exercise was inspired by Michelle Horman (see her exercise in this volume), who often adapted her theatre-based vocal methods to free up the voice in a therapeutic setting. The messa-di-voce component of this exercise came from observing a workshop by Sharon Freed at the Voice Symposium in 2007. By mirroring the volume of the voice with the height of the arm swings, this exercise can be particularly successful in establishing a clear connection between projected voice, the dynamics of breath support, and postural energy.

Editors' Note: Compare this exercise to Horman's Arm Swing Warm-Up in this volume. Here, Gherson's exercise targets loud voice production, whereas Horman's exercise focuses upon general body-voice connection and breath support.

Overview

The progression of moving from soft to loud voice production is visually modeled by the height of a rhythmic swinging of the arms. The swing is coordinated with trills, hums, or syllables; a low swing matching the softer phonation and a high arm swing accompanying the louder voice. The larger, more effortful movement of the high swing can engage a greater sense of respiratory support for loud voicing. When building up from a soft to loud voice, the client experiences the shifting dynamics of energy required for each loudness level.

The Exercise

1. Set up for the arm swing by placing one foot in front of the other to provide a base for rocking back and forth with the swing of the arms. Swing your arms while moving your hips forward and back in the direction of the swing. Your swings should be rhythmic and relaxed. To prepare for vocalizing,

inhale when your arms swing back and exhale when you throw them forward.

2. Begin with a low swing, producing a moderately soft production of a voiced trill, hum, or syllable when your arms swing in front of you. Repeat this 5 to 10 times.

3. Expand the swing of your arms to shoulder height. Repeat the same vocalization with a louder voice (consistent with conversational loudness level). Continue to feel the connection with the movement of the swing.

4. Finally, swing your arms fully up overhead. Take time for a deeper breath with a steady stance. Use a projected voice, imagining that you are "throwing" the sound in a high and far reaching arch.

5. Return to moderate loudness and finally softer voice, bringing the arm swing down accordingly.

6. Carryover can include /h/ initial words starting with a soft "ho," moving to a modal "hey," and projecting the voice on the word "high!"

Breath Sensitivity Training

Martin L. Spencer

Purposes

- To increase client awareness of the contribution of breathing to phonation
- To regulate efficient transglottal airflow for phonation
- To facilitate diaphragmatic/abdominal involvement during breathing, and limit neck/clavicular tension
- To moderate somatic-emotional manifestations of anxiety and stress.

Origin

This series of exploratory exercises has ancient roots and is currently espoused in a wide range of disciplines from theatre and healing to athletics and religion. Various approaches to lower abdominal breathing were taught to me by David Smith and Colin Bernhardt, talented pedagogues in the experimental Music Theater Studio Ensemble at the Banff School of Fine Arts, and Richard Armstrong of the Roy Hart Theater. These series of "breathwork" workshops were designed to explore the psyche through emotional release from the intellect, leading to liberation of the "dramatic self." An interesting facet of this training focused on *metaphysical color breathing*, which addresses release of mental stress and its negative effects on the body.

It is surmised in theatre, music, and meditation techniques that breath is intimately connected with "life source energy," and that access to the potential of lower abdominal breathing is generally a learned or rediscovered phenomenon. This type of "out there" thinking is commonly addressed within the dramatic arts. Although many voice therapists may not be acquainted with these approaches, they may have some relevance for therapists interested in a holistic interventional approach to rehabilitation. Interestingly, I've never had a voice client who was skeptical of this type of work after rehabilitative exposure.

Overview

Breathing techniques (the Basic Exercise and the Windspread) provide an excellent starting point for voice rehabilitation. Voice clients often focus excessively on the sound of the voice and ignore the subtler kinesthetic feedback of the breathing system. Therefore, this exercise begins with examination of breathing without voice. The sequence may be expanded with progressive relaxation and visualization.

Note: Throughout these exercises, the therapist models the target behavior and demonstrates potentially incorrect behavior.

The Exercises

The Basic Exercise

Gauge upper chest position as being neither artificially elevated nor depressed. To monitor respiratory movement, and after gaining the client's permission, place your hand over your client's hand, which is resting palm-in on the lower belly. To similar purpose, another hand may be placed over the small of the back. Maintain this position for Steps one through three.

1. Stand erect, allowing the spinal column to elongate and decompress. The goal is a free sensation in the neck, shoulders, hips, and limbs.
2. While exhaling, feel the inward-directed movement of the abdomen. ("The lungs are deflating like a balloon that will suck in your gut.")
3. Inhale deeply through your nose; allow the inspiration to dilate the nares and nasopharynx. Avoid superfluous upper chest involvement. Imagery such as slowly filling your lungs from the bottom up or expanding all around your beltline may help establish abdominal control.
4. Blow out through gently pursed lips, allow the cheeks to inflate. Exhale in one sustained pulse, seemingly driven by elastic contraction of the torso.
5. Aim at 10 breath cycles of gentle, energized breathing. Pause to allow recovery from possible lightheadedness. For home practice, the goal is three sets of 10 cycles performed three times a day.

A common tendency is to fully inflate the lungs before the arms have reached the 180° endpoint. Direction to move the arms like a fuel gauge needle ("¼ . . . ½ . . . ¾ . . . full") may help pace the client appropriately.

Windspread

This exercise consists of preparatory elements of Tai Chi in combination with movements from dance and vocal training. An advanced variation on the Basic Exercise, it addresses breathing, freely energized posture, and outward-directed "energy flow" that may compel listener attention during teaching or public speaking.

I use the image of arms representing the needle in a car's fuel gauge, coordinating arm movement with lung volume: arms in front of the body represents empty lungs, whereas arms at either side represents full. This imagery and accompanying movement tends to slow the cycle and promote awareness of the breath control mechanism.

1. Stand with your feet parallel and a shoulder-width apart. Direct decompression upward from the base of the spine through the cervical vertebrae (think of a rising "current of energy"). Relax the hips and slightly bend the knees so that the torso is buoyant. Elevate and extend the arms directly in front of the torso, with hands facing the ground and fingers extended. Relax the shoulders.
2. Rotate the arms laterally, parallel to the ground, and coordinate breathing so that you reach maximal inhalation when your arms are outstretched to 180°. Think of treading water with your hands and thumbs naturally rotating downward. Do not overly inhale.
3. In a fluid rebounding movement, return the arms slowly to the initial frontal position with hands now rotated upward and fingers gently spread (treading water again). Exhale smoothly via pursed but not clenched lips during this movement.
4. Cycle through five repetitions. Make sure that the movements are smooth and unrushed.

Matwork: A Progressive Relaxation

I was introduced to matwork by Colin Bernhardt, a gentle but powerfully energizing soul, during theatre training at the Banff Center. I believe that progressive relaxation exercises are extremely valuable in the treatment of somatic hyperfunction and anxiety, common factors that inhibit vocal release. In this type of work, it is ideal to have a mat which can be rolled up and kept in your therapy area. The advantage of working with a prone client is that the extensive skeletal musculature that maintains an erect posture is able to relax. This relaxation allows a client to focus on the subtlety of breath movement within the torso.

1. Lie with your back on the mat with outstretched legs. Arms may lie to the side or with hands resting on your belly. Induce a pull upward through the cervical vertebrae. Your neck and chin should flex neither upward nor downward. Eyes should be closed.
2. Initiate an internal scan by sensing foot position and heel weight on the mat. Pause for proprioceptive feedback. Rising

When the client is focused on the neck, you may need to manually elongate the neck and reposition the head.

through the body, direct your awareness to the weight and position of calves, knees, thighs, and hips. Allow each component to relax by "melting into the floor" and reposition through the pull of gravity. Pause at each level to experience full sensation of component weight into the mat.

3. As you continue to sense the weight of your body on the mat, focus on the small of the back. If you can, you may press the lumbar vertebrae into the mat and then release the area to assume a natural curvature. Continue the slow routing of awareness up through the spine and pause in the thoracic region between the scapulae. Feel the weight of the shoulders, and direct the scapulae to displace laterally, away from the central spinal tug. Direct your consciousness into the tips of the shoulders and downward through the upper arms, elbows, lower arms, wrists, hands, and finally into the release of fingers and thumbs. Pause. Move awareness back up through the arms and medially through the clavicles. Pause at the base of the neck and scan upward to feel the weight of the head, heavy on the mat. The contact area of your head with the mat is small (the size of a silver dollar). Focus now on the curvature of the nape of the neck. Move the scan upward, and curl over the top of the head. Relax the muscles of the forehead, around the eyebrows, eyes, cheeks, jaw, and lips.

On completion of each set of exercises, pause for a moment and then engage the client in reflective conversation about his or her observations.

4. Your body should now be in a state of "purposeful repose." Now direct your attention to the movement of cool air in through the mouth (if the jaw is relaxed then the mouth may instinctively open) and into the pharynx. Try to sense where the cool room air becomes warmed to body temperature in the deep pharynx, and continue with the ingress of warmed breath down to the bottom of the lungs. Allow your breathing to settle into an abdominally centered pattern and experience the flow of breath in the midst of deep relaxation. After a minute or so, open your eyes and become attuned to the sounds around you, perhaps a clock ticking or the noise of a computer fan. Rest momentarily in this state of heightened sensory awareness until finally you roll over onto your side, curl your legs, and make your way up to sitting or standing.

Chromatherapy: Visualization

When the client has reached a state of readiness induced by progressive relaxation, then direct the breathing cycle to nasal inspiration and gentle, oral, pursed lip exhalation.

1. Close your eyes and inhale and exhale an imaginary "white mist." (A variant is to imagine the incoming mist flowing down the ventral torso, and the outgoing mist flowing up the dorsum.) After several such cycles, gently hold the inspired breath/mist

deep in the torso for five seconds while imagining the white mist (alone) percolating up through the spine and whirling around within the cranium. The mist should then be dispelled with moderately vigorous breath exhalation. Repeat through several cycles.

2. Next, visualize a sequence in which the white mist is spinning inside your head. It dissolves anxiety or emotional tension, thus becoming a mottled gray. The solute-laden mist is then vigorously expelled with the breath through pursed lips to a region above the body. Work through several cycles of "in with the new and out with the old." At this point, you may introduce color variants, with the idea that a "pure" color (such as yellow, red, or blue) carries away impurities in the form of a more complex color, such as burnt orange, purple, or brown. (Some clients with a history of emotional pain find it helpful to use an image of blood red mist transforming into the multihued darkness of a bruise.) Complete the exercise by returning to the initial cycling of white mist and finally colorless breath with opened eyes.

I Like to Move It! Move It! Kinesthetically Speaking

Ashley Paseman

Purposes

- To achieve good speech-breathing support.
- To release musculoskeletal tension.
- To initiate voice consistently with coordinated airflow.
- To achieve and maintain appropriate speaking pitch.

Origin

These exercises were inspired by attending conference workshops for the acting voice, and being forced to participate outside of my comfort zone. As a medically based speech-language pathologist, my treatment approach had often focused on structured, evidence-based hygiene and symptomatic therapy. However, I came to realize the potential for voice improvement that can be achieved through kinesthetically based training. These exercises have been a helpful addition to my eclectic therapy approach, and often yield terrific results.

Overview

These exercises begin with some simple stretches and then progress to adding phonation coordinated with rhythmic body movement. The goal is to capitalize on the energy that is produced with body movement to help achieve a clear, fluid speaking voice.

The Exercise

I. Stretching and Breathing

1. Start with some generalized stretching to warm up the body and release tension. These warm-ups can include any of the following:

   - Shoulder rolls in one direction and then the other
   - Swinging your arms in circles, alternating left, then right
   - Lifting your arms overhead and leaning to the right, then left
   - Rocking your hips back to front and around in circles.

2. Now, we want to position the body to feel the breath. Starting from a standing position, slump over like a rag doll. As you are slumped over, pay attention to movement in your body as you inhale and exhale. When you inhale, feel the lower abdominal muscles move, and feel the expansion of your lower back. As you exhale, try to let the ribs close slowly instead of collapsing rapidly.

3. When you have established this connection between your breathing and movements of the abdomen and rib cage, on an inhalation slowly roll up from the slumped position until you are standing upright and then exhale.

> If the client is having difficulty achieving the target sensations in the upright position, have the client lie down, squat, or get on his or her hands and knees. Again, the focus is on feeling the abdominal muscles moving out and the lower back expanding during inhalation, and then in the opposite direction for exhalation.

Ok, now let's move it!

II. Swing Voice

These steps aim to connect the body to the breath and the voice while moving. Keep in mind that we are targeting fluid motion and whole body connection with the sound.

1. Start by swaying (rocking) side to side from one foot to another, shifting your weight.

2. Now add swinging arms as you sway (rock) from one foot to the other. Swing both of your arms in a pendular motion across your body, parallel to the sway as you shift your weight. Continue swaying (rocking) side to side with the arms swinging in a fluid motion.

3. Now add voicing as you swing by counting from 1 to 10. Start first with a single swing for each count: swing "one," swing "two," swing "three," swing "four," swing "five." The voice should be produced with a slightly elevated pitch in a "singsong" style, with upward inflection as you swing the voice "up" with your arms for each count. Then you can speed up the count and grouping of numbers from 1 to 10: swing "one-two," swing "three-four," swing "five-six," swing "seven-eight," swing "nine-ten."

4. Once you are able to produce the body movement coordinated with the voicing easily and freely, repeat the exercise but now speak the numbers without the swing gesture. Recall the sensation of easy rhythm, however, and maintain a similar energy in the voice.

5. Now use the side-to-side rocking and arm swinging with short, simple phrases, then fade the body movement as you repeat the utterances and maintain the energy. Continue with more complex utterances.

III. *March to the Beat*

1. March in place using a steady beat, swinging your arms back and forth in time to your marching feet. Make sure that you use low (abdominal) breathing while you march.

2. As you march, add an accented *staccato*-like clipped counting 1–2–3–4! Maintain good speech-breathing support.

3. Make the transition fairly rapidly into actually marching around the room, with the same staccato-style counting, and extending the length of the counting sequence to 10.

4. Once the connection between breath, movement, and voice is well established, alternate between marching with the count and standing for a count, as in march "1–2–3–4," stand "5–6–7–8," march "1–2–3–4," stand "5–6–7–8."

5. Next, transition into standing in place and counting, maintaining the same coordination of breath and energy while speaking.

6. Move progressively into short utterances, phrases, and sentences. Physical cues should gradually be faded out while maintaining the goal of a clear and fluid speaking voice that is driven by the coordinated breath and energy.

Play with the speaking pitch, by "vocally bobbing" up and down, alternating between two pitches, separated by thirds, fifths, or even an octave in the client's middle voice register.

"One" (lower pitch/ "Two" (higher pitch)

"Three" (lower pitch)/ "Four" (higher pitch)

"Five (lower pitch)/ "Six" (higher pitch)

For those clients who need extra help moving the voice upward, it may be helpful to have the client pair the marching with accented 'punching' with the arms to the beat. Some sample patterns are as follows.

Rhythmically punching both arms overhead

Rhythmically alternating punching left and right arms to the front of the body

Rhythmically punching both arms outward, starting at chest level and gradually moving upward until the arms are directly overhead, and then progressing back downward.

Alexander-Based Vocal Therapy: With a Little Help from Carl Stough

Joan Lader and Jessica Wolf

Purposes

- To increase awareness of the contribution of the entire body to breathing and voice production.
- To encourage efficient voice production with minimal effort through use of Alexander technique.

Origin

The Alexander Technique is a method of movement reeducation that teaches dynamic postural balance and efficient breathing coordination. The technique was developed by F. M. Alexander, who was a Shakespearean actor, famous for his dramatic recitations. The popular story is reported that, during performances, he noticed that his voice was becoming hoarse with increasing vocal demands and on a recurring basis. Doctors advised him to rest his voice, but as soon as he began to use it again, the problem would recur. Alexander decided to be his own therapist and began observing the manner in which his body was involved when producing sound. He identified a pattern of habitual misuse that was causing him to restrict his breath, and discovered a new way of movement in which the head balances on the spine, resulting in a freer and more efficient manner of speech.

The field of breathing re-education has also benefited from the contributions of Carl Stough. Stough's unique discovery identified the diaphragm as the primary muscle of breathing and demonstrated that although the diaphragm functions involuntarily, its movement can be influenced by voluntary motor behaviors.

It is our belief that an individual's faulty movement patterns affect the breathing system and may be the underlying cause of many hyperfunctional as well as hypofunctional voice disorders. The body and voice are deeply connected. In order for the voice to work effectively, the body must be freely balanced, with good breath support to activate the vocal folds.

Overview

These exercises are based on the principles of Alexander Technique. The exercises are performed by the client in three positions, beginning with the semisupine, and proceeding to sitting, and then to standing positions. Throughout the process, the therapist provides hands-on guidance and encourages the client to remain mindful of the whole body.

Five repetitions of each cycle should be performed. Each step is complete on its own. Always begin with the exhale. Inhalation will become reflexive.

The Exercises

I. Semisupine

The Preparation

The therapist guides the client as follows:

1. Lie on your back, with your knees bent and your feet placed flat on the floor, approximately hip-width apart. The head is supported by books, and the hands rest on the abdomen. Taking time to lie down and release muscular tension that has built up over the course of a day gently realigns the spine, re-establishes connections among all parts of the torso and body, and thus encourages improved breathing. The books prevent the head from collapsing back, exaggerating the curve of the neck and shortening the spine, constricting the throat and the breath.
2. Notice if you tend to stiffen your neck. Think of freeing the neck to allow your torso to release back toward the floor as your back widens. Direct your attention to releasing the muscles. Don't press your lower back against the floor, but allow the spine to retain its natural curves.
3. Think about the head releasing away from the top of the spine. Note that the spine actually ends at the level of your ears and behind your nose. Your neck lengthens up behind your jaw.

4. Begin with an exhalation: gently release the breath and allow it to return naturally. You are not actively taking a breath. Trust the breath to come back after you exhale (recoil).

5. Feel the subtle, three-dimensional movement of the back, spine, and torso as you breathe easily. Notice the mobility of your ribs as your back releases into length and width, releasing jaw and neck tension. Do not move your ribs in order to breathe; allow your ribs to move as a result of the breath moving in and out of your body.

The Vocal Tasks

The client now begins the exercises, guided by the therapist's instructions. Each exercise begins with an exhalation. We proceed from simple extended exhalations through increasingly challenging vocal production. In each exercise, the inhalation should occur as a reflexive response to completion of the exhalation, allowing the exercise to be repeated with the next exhalation.

Silent "La": Allow the tip of the tongue to wag or flap as you mouth a silent "la, la, la." This encourages a complete exhalation and a more natural, reflexive inhalation in response. Go to the end of the breath but do not force it. Imagine that the breath can fuel the length of the spine during both inhalation and exhalation.

Silent Count: Silently count from 1 to 10 using your articulators. Do not "enunciate" with effort; tension interferes with the release of the breath and disturbs the rhythmic return of the inhale.

Counting Aloud: Begin with an audible count of 5. Once the next breath arrives, count to 10. Increase the count gradually as you repeat the exercise.

Whispered /ɑ/: With the tip of the tongue resting behind the lower teeth and the mouth opening, whisper an extended /ɑ:/.

Sung /ɑ/: Sing the vowel /ɑ:/ on any comfortable pitch, stopping when it can no longer be sustained without effort. When the exhalation is complete, allow the breath to return before singing /ɑ/ again.

Variations: Repeat the whispered /ɑ:/ and sung /ɑ:/ with a long /i:/, or a combination of vowels. The same protocol can be practiced using rote speech, such as days of the week, months of the year, or nursery rhymes, for example.

II. Sitting

Sitting can be very challenging. Slumping or collapsing into the chair puts a great deal of pressure on the joints of the spine and can spell disaster for the lower back. However, overcorrecting this problem by pulling up in front causes other problems: constricting the back, tightening the torso, and holding the breath. Crossing the legs is equally threatening, as it encourages both tightening and collapse.

The Preparation

The therapist guides the client to sit on a hard, straight-backed chair using one of the following two methods.

1. Sit on your sitting bones close to the front edge with both of your feet on the floor. Let your weight release down. The chair will support your weight. Think of your head leading forward and up and allow your torso to lengthen and widen. Your muscles will develop and learn to support your spine.
2. Sit all the way back in the seat and use the back of the chair for support. Allow the sitting bones to release toward the chair and let your feet rest flat on the floor.

The Vocal Tasks

Now the therapist guides the client through the vocal tasks as described above in Section I Semisupine.

III. Standing

Finally, the vocal tasks are repeated in a dynamic standing posture, "thinking up" without stiffening—a combination of stability and mobility. Good breath support does *not* consist of drawing in the abdominal muscles or tightening any part of the body; such tension will close the throat and restrict the breath. Instead, allowing the torso to lengthen and widen helps release the ribs and the throat, which is essential for the breath and voice to work well.

The Preparation

The therapist guides the client as follows:

1. Release the neck muscles from any tension, so that your head can ease up off the top of your spine.
2. The head must balance freely at the top of the spine so that the whole body can fully expand. The back should feel firm but not tense. This state of coordination allows you to be responsive to yourself and the environment around you.
3. Lengthen your entire spine toward your head and let your heels release down toward the ground. Let your feet receive the full weight of your entire body. Avoid locking your knees or clenching in the buttocks.
4. Think of your shoulders moving apart from each other, releasing any habitual tension in the chest and shoulder girdle. The motion of your breath should be experienced throughout your body, stimulating you to maintain your full length and width.

The Vocal Tasks

Now the therapist guides the client through the vocal tasks as described above in Section I Semisupine.

Chapter 7

ARTICULATORY FREEDOM

Traditionally, in our graduate school training, in relation to the topic of articulation, we are primed to think about speech sound errors. And when we concern ourselves with voice production, our initial thoughts are of the larynx, the breath support system, and the supraglottal region, particularly the activity of the false vocal folds. But as we gain experience in working with voice therapy clients (and particularly for those therapists who have a background in singing or acting) we come to realize that articulation—the movement of the tongue, the lips, and the mandible—affects resonance and breathing, and therefore it affects the effort and efficiency with which we vibrate our vocal folds and produce voice. And so attention to articulation becomes an integral component of our therapy efforts.

The techniques we use encompass, first, increasing the client's awareness of articulatory movement and its effect on voice production. (See the discussion in the introductory chapter of this book about the effect of self-awareness on change in motor behaviors.) We may then distort our client's articulation, temporarily through chewing movements or exaggerated tongue postures, toward the ultimate goal of overall balanced vocal production. We may then fade out the exaggerated articulatory postures while maintaining its positive effects of increased freedom of movement and improved resonance. And finally, we may seek to transfer the newly learned skills to many other communicative contexts.

Five exercises are included in this section. Haskell's *Articulatory Awareness* guides the client in an exploration of self-awareness of the kinesthetics of articulatory movement and the changes in those movements as a function of speech rate and linguistic content. Two more exercises, Haskell's *Chewing Method* and Ma's *Chewing Technique*, both incorporate the classic Chewing Method in various ways. This approach capitalizes on the freedom of movement that occurs naturally during the vegetative act of chewing, imbuing the spoken phrase with a similar freedom of movement that enhances the production of voice. Schneider, in *Tongue-Out Phonation*, helps the client to release excessive tongue tension, and thereby facilitate low breathing and forward resonance, by positioning the tongue far forward in the mouth while practicing a hierarchy of voicing tasks. The tongue is then slowly brought back to a normal position during talking, but now ideally without the accompanying hyperfunction. Fava and Oliveira, in *Tongue Teaser*, also address tongue tension, and propose repetitive production of the syllable "gla," with the tongue tip lowered for the "l" sound, as a way of reducing tongue tension and supraglottic constriction.

Beyond this chapter, you will find that many of the other exercises in this book can be adapted readily for the client who demonstrates excessive oral articulatory hyperfunction. Try having your clients "chew" some of the other exercises, or place their tongue far forward, or simply increase their awareness of the movement of their articulators.

Articulatory Awareness

John Haskell

Purposes

- To increase awareness of articulatory movements and contacts.
- To increase articulatory flexibility and precision.
- To facilitate front-focus resonance.

Origin

These exercises are part of a broader program for voice therapy that I call Balanced Vocal Energy. The goal of the program is to direct vocal effort away from the larynx to three specific areas of vocal energy: speech breathing, speech melody, and articulatory movement. Increasing articulatory awareness and control in voice production is a way of enabling the client to monitor and maintain the balance of vocal effort. It also helps the client produce a forward focus of resonance.

Overview

The main goal of these simple exercises is awareness. The therapist must stress that the purpose is not exaggeration of articulation, but, rather, awareness of movements and contacts of the articulators. (A key factor in the exercises is that increased attention to articulatory movements and contacts typically causes the client to display more jaw movement and more oral space while speaking, often a goal in voice therapy.) The therapist should also check for comfortable breathing and relaxed speech rhythm.

Exercise 1 deals mainly with the lip sounds *p*, *b*, *m*. Exercise 2 deals with *w* and the tongue-tip sound *n*, which is useful for its durational and resonance potential. Exercise 3 is included to increase general awareness of articulatory movements in the flow of speech. Each of these exercises should be performed two or three times. Exercise 4 is an extension of the process into conversational speech. Exercises 1 through 3 may be performed with the client's eyes closed for tactile-kinesthetic feedback, or with the use of a mirror for visual feedback. After each exercise, the therapist should question the client about the sensations of movements and contacts.

The Exercises

1. September–October
Say the last four months of the year twice, quickly, with your eyes closed. As you say the months, concentrate on your lips. Take a full breath before you start. You may also do the exercise with the months February–May.

2. One-Hundred-and-One
Count from 101 to 112, two numbers at a time at a comfortable pace. Take a relaxed breath between each pair of numbers. Feel the tip of the tongue tap the gum ridge every time you articulate an /n/. Feel your lips become rounded as you produce the /w/ sound for the beginning of the number "one."

> One-hundred-and-one-one-hundred-and-two [*breath*] . . .
> one-hundred-and-eleven-one-hundred-and-twelve

Count again, three numbers (later, four numbers) on a breath. Go a little faster; see if you can still feel the movements.

3. 7/11
Take a medium breath and count smoothly from 1 to 7. Take another breath and count from 5 to 11. As you are counting, be aware of overall movement of the lips and tongue. In the first phrase (1–7), focus on your lips, with special attention to /f/ and /v/; in the second phrase (5–11), focus on your tongue tip, with special attention to each /n/. Repeat with relaxed breathing and rhythmic flow.

> 1 – 2 – 3 – 4 – 5 – 6 – 7 //
> 5 – 6 – 7 – 8 – 9 – 10 – 11

4. Carryover
Place your fingers lightly on the sides of your jaw. Talk briefly about three things that you did today. While you are talking, concentrate on the movements of your jaw, lips, and tongue.

The carryover part of the exercise may be extended as far as the client and therapist deem necessary, with more complex content in monologue or dialogue speech. In dialogue speech, the client and therapist may watch each other's articulatory movements as a visual stimulus to increase self-monitoring.

The Chewing Method

John Haskell

Purpose

■ To establish a balance of muscular tension in vocal production, thereby minimizing vocal hyperfunction.

Origin

The Chewing Method was developed in the 1930s by Emil Froeschels, an otolaryngologist, who was seeking a holistic approach for treatment of speech and voice disorders. He considered that, for primitive human beings, speaking and chewing were essentially the same function. Therefore, he reasoned, if a client chews normally, then he or she should be able to re-establish normal phonation. The client would move from vocalized chewing, free of linguistic constraints, to a "chewing attitude" with language production. The chewing method was widely used in Europe and the United States during the mid-20th century (Froeschels, 1952). Interest waned when the original practitioners were no longer alive and as the field of voice therapy expanded.

I learned the chewing method from Friedrich S. Brodnitz, M.D., a well-known otolaryngologist who was a colleague of Froeschels. I have found the method to be a quick, effective approach for many clients, particularly those willing to make exaggerated oral movements and sounds. Actors and singers are especially responsive to this method, as are young children. It can be presented as a behavioral approach (without the underlying philosophy), that is, with a set of behaviors, appropriately reinforced and practiced within a strict schedule. The description below includes adaptations that I have made over the years.

> I have found that the Chewing Method, if done correctly, is actually a form of resonant voice therapy. It places the focus of the tone forward, establishes a smooth breathing and legato flow, and reinforces the front focus with articulatory flexibility, thereby minimizing vocal effort.

Overview

The method can be presented in three basic lessons. The first three steps below constitute Lesson I, and should take no more than a minute. The sequence is repeated several times in the session. The therapist should demonstrate each of the steps, chew with the client if necessary, and make sure that the client's vocalizations do not become too nasal. Lessons II and III, Steps 4 to 6, can be presented subsequently in several sessions over a period of a month.

Note: This exercise is contraindicated for clients with temporo-mandibular joint dysfunction.

The Exercise

Some clients may need a piece of bread or cracker to initiate the exercise.

1. Chew vigorously with your mouth closed. Keep your tongue active, and breathe in a relaxed manner. Gradually add short stretches of humming, as if you are enjoying something tasty.

2. Now chew vigorously with your mouth open. Keep your tongue active, as if you are moving food and saliva around in your mouth. Remember to breathe comfortably. Add humming, and move on to yum-yum-yum (several times) with strong, forward tongue movement.

3. Continue chewing vigorously and count to 7 (or say the days of the week). Speak quickly, and don't try to articulate clearly. Concentrate on chewing.

4. After you have had a few days of practicing Steps 1 to 3, you should try the counting with three levels of chewing: (a) vigorous chewing, (b) moderate chewing, and (c) minimal chewing or "think-chew."

5. When you are able to move easily from one level to another, read a short paragraph at each of the three levels. You can also apply the three levels to other material that you know, such as the Pledge of Allegiance and nursery rhymes.

6. A good way to apply chewing to conversational speech is with telephone calls. (If you chew too vigorously during the call, no one will see you.) You should try a few calls in the therapy session, role-playing first.

Chewing Technique: Speak with an "Open Mouth"

Estella Ma

Purposes

- To reduce generalized hyperfunction in the vocal tract.
- To improve loudness and vocal quality by increasing oral cavity size during speaking.

Origin

This exercise combines the chewing technique with a focus on an open mouth. The use of chewing as a vocal facilitative technique for hyperfunctional voice disorders was first proposed by Froeschels (1952) and has been described widely in voice textbooks (Boone, McFarlane, & Von Berg, 2005; Colton, Casper, & Leonard, 2006) (See Haskell's exercise on chewing in this chapter for more details on its origin.). The additional focus on the open mouth addresses a common problem of jaw tension and limited oral range of motion during speaking.

Overview

Because chewing is a vegetative function that involves jaw movement, when a speaker applies chewing to speaking, it may result in increased oral cavity space, and stronger oral resonance. I have found that a combination of the chewing method with a focus on open mouth works well with clients who demonstrate limited oral movement while speaking.

Note: As a preliminary step, have the client clench lightly his or her teeth to feel the masseter muscles contract and release. This action helps the client to increase muscle awareness and jaw tension. If the client reports jaw joint discomfort during this exercise, discontinue, and consider referral to a dentist.

The Exercise

1. Sustain /ɑ/ for approximately three seconds as you view your face in the mirror. Note the amount of opening of your mouth. Repeat the sustained vowel, this time opening your mouth a little more. Make sure that your teeth are separated by at least

Editors' Note:

Compare the differences between Ma's, Haskell's, and Schneider's chewing exercises. Here, Ma focuses on the open mouth from the start of the chewing and retains the focus of mouth aperture throughout the exercise. Haskell begins with a closed mouth and then, as the client moves to the chew combined with speech, the focus remains on the chewing. Also, Ma incorporates the chewing into phrases with the bilabial glide and nasals, whereas Haskell focuses on blending chewing into rote speech. Schneider uses chewing as a means to achieve frontal oral resonance, and maintains the client's focus on the sensation of resonance throughout the exercise, rather than the chewing movements. The different presentations of a similar technique provide a good demonstration of how a basic exercise can be approached in different manners to address the needs of the individual client.

one finger's width. Practice sustaining the vowel so that you can easily produce the sound with a relaxed jaw.

2. Now start a relaxed, gentle chewing motion, approximately one chew per second, opening your mouth as you did for the sustained vowel. Keep the chewing continuous, with a smooth vertical motion, slightly exaggerating movement of the lips.

3. Add soft phonation, producing a sound like "yum-yum." Continue to feel relaxed as you produce the yum-yum, and allow your voice to emerge clearly with strong oral resonance. Check to make sure that you are opening your mouth as you chew to at least one finger's width.

4. Practice with monosyllabic words starting with the glide /w/ or nasal /m/. Feel the yum-yum merge into the words, exaggerating slightly the /w/ or /m/.

   For example:

   (chewing) yum-yum—why

   (chewing) yum-yum—way

   (chewing) yum-yum—mine

   (chewing) yum-yum—may

5. Practice with disyllabic words. Chew yum-yum and then blend into the first syllable. The chewing is faded as you say the second syllable.

   For example:

   (chewing) yum-yum—why me (or wireless, waving, warning)

6. Practice yum-yum with words starting with other consonants, and then progress to simple daily phrases. Chew yum-yum, blending the chew into the first syllable of the phrase, and fading the chew throughout the remainder of the phrase.

   For example:

   (chewing) yum-yum—Open the door, please.

   (chewing) yum-yum—Good morning.

7. Repeat Steps 4 through 6 without the initial chew. Mentally rehearse the sensation of the chewing. Check for any jaw tension, and allow minimal chewing movement.

Tongue-Out Phonation

Sarah L. Schneider

Purposes

- To minimize tongue retraction, base of tongue tension, and jaw tension during phonation.
- To increase speech breathing support.
- To elicit increased oral resonance through wider oral-pharyngeal space and emphasis on front-of-the-mouth articulation.

Origin

I began using this exercise to decrease base of tongue tension/tongue retraction during phonation, after observing a colleague using a variation of this exercise in voice therapy.

Overview

The exercise begins by establishing relaxed abdominal breathing with the tongue released over the lower lip. During this quiet breathing it may become apparent that the tongue retracts on inhalation and/or exhalation. This retraction movement should be decreased. Phonation is then added beginning with a sigh and then progressing to more complex utterances. Ultimately, when utterances can be produced consistently with minimal tongue retraction, the phonatory task can be repeated alternating tongue out and tongue in, gradually fading the use of tongue-out phonation.

Note: An open breath begins each task in this exercise.

> Practice the open breath. The open breath is open-mouth breathing that promotes a sensation of an open, relaxed throat (increased oral-pharyngeal space) during inhalation and an absence of muscular hyperfunction. The jaw should be in a released position, allowing space in between the tongue and upper incisors, and the tongue should remain quiet. (Avoid retraction on inhalation.). Low ("abdominal") breathing should be used throughout.

The Exercise

1. Take an open breath, keeping the tongue relaxed over the lower lip and practice initiating voicing with a sighed /ɑ/. It is important to avoid tongue retraction during both inhalation and phonation.
2. Use a labial consonant while closing the lips around the tongue to articulate the sound /mɑ:/ or /bɑ:/. Use of these consonants should increase the sensation of forward/oral resonance. Complete a series of /mɑmɑ/ on various vowels (such as /mimi/ and /momo/) to prevent tongue retraction on all vowels. Guard

> If the client is having difficulty achieving an open breath in a relaxed manner, a yawn may facilitate the sensation of increased oral-pharyngeal space. Cue the client to produce a yawn inhalation, which should elicit a dropped jaw, raised palate, and widened pharynx. Alternatively, cue the client to produce a hidden or stifled yawn, with the breath taken in through the nose, the lips gently closed, and the jaw released.

against holding the jaw rigidly, making sure to allow it to move freely during articulation. Practice until the behavior is well established.

3. Now say words and phrases with the tongue-out position. Remember to maintain a relaxed tongue over the lower lip, and a freely moving jaw. Begin each utterance with the tongue out and an open breath and continue to maintain good speech-breathing support. Practice with a variety of utterances until the behavior is well-established.

4. Now alternate tongue-out and tongue-in phonation. Take an open breath while the tongue is protruded and say a word or phrase. Bring the tongue in, take an open breath, and say the same utterance. The vocal ease and quality that are achieved with the tongue-out phonation should be maintained when the tongue is brought in.

5. Continue to increase the complexity of utterances, progressing to paragraph reading and conversation, alternating tongue out and tongue in as needed. As the ability to maintain the sensation of increased oral-pharyngeal space and forward resonance increases, the tongue-out phonation may be faded, using it only at the beginning of paragraph reading or conversation. Ultimately, the tongue out phonation can be used only as needed to regain the target resonance.

Tongue Teaser

Gaetano Fava and Gisele Oliveira

Purposes

- To release back of the tongue tension during phonation
- To increase awareness of compensatory tongue control
- To ease production of low and high frequencies
- To reduce supraglottic constriction.

Origin

We were introduced to the basic principles of this exercise during singing classes with Jeanie LoVetri, singing teacher, founder and director of The Voice Workshop™, and creator of Somatic Voicework™.

Overview

This exercise particularly benefits clients with vocal hyperfunction —presenting with vocal tract constriction and compensatory tongue movement during extreme vocal range production—and clients who are also singers. The aim of this exercise is to produce the "GLA" sound, an articulatory consonant cluster, with the back of the tongue touching the palate, rather than with the tip of the tongue. Typically, the /l/ from this cluster is produced by placing the tip of the tongue against the alveolar ridge and lowering its central portion. During the performance of this exercise, however, the tip of the tongue remains anchored behind the lower incisors and the sound is produced by elevating the back of the tongue against the posterior section of the hard palate. By bringing the tongue in this forward position, the larynx elevates, the ventricular folds open, and supraglottic constriction decreases.

Note: The therapist should walk the client through the exercise step-by-step and model it until client can perform the exercise accurately. The sound produced must be light, soft, and effortless. Particular attention should be paid to the following aspects: (1) The tongue tip should not move; (2) The jaw should not be fixed. It should move loosely with the production of the sound; and (3) Compensatory nasal resonance, devoicing of the cluster, and tense vocal quality should all be avoided.

For each aspect that the client has difficulty producing successfully (devoicing, nasality), cue the client one aspect at a time until mastered before moving on to the next. Voice breaks are not negative and are expected during higher pitch production.

This technique can function as a preparatory exercise prior to engaging the client in other vocal tasks designed to work towards connected speech, such as resonant voice or vocal function exercises.

The Exercise

1. Place the tip of the tongue behind the lower incisors and start producing the "GLA" repetitively, with a moderate speech rate, in comfortable pitch, soft loudness, and flow/breathy phonation. The tip of the tongue must be anchored throughout the entire exercise. The jaw must be loose and moving with each articulated sound. Repeat this step until you are able to produce a clear, constant, effortless, and breathy "GLA."

2. When you are successful with production of the basic exercise, begin introducing pitch variations, extending the range continuously over time and practice. Vary the exercise from single tones to scales of thirds, fifths, and octaves.

Chapter 8

TEACHING LOUD VOICE PRODUCTION

Under what circumstances would we want to teach a client how to talk loudly in a healthy and efficient manner? Perhaps it is easier to answer the other side of the question: For which clients would we *not* want to teach loud voice production? Certainly loud speaking is contraindicated in cases of phonotrauma. And a client who rarely, if ever, uses a loud voice would have little need for such exercises. But consider the elementary school teacher with vocal fold nodules who takes turns supervising the lunchroom and the playground, or the waiter who works in a noisy restaurant. Consider the shop steward with muscle tension dysphonia who must converse with employees on the floor of a busy manufacturing plant, or the mother with young children. And finally, consider the client who converses frequently with a family member who is hearing impaired, or the actor whose voice must carry to the last row of the balcony. In fact, many of our clients need to use a loud voice on a daily basis. Rather than admonishing the client to avoid loud voice use, it is often more practical to teach the client how to achieve a loud voice in a healthy manner.

The five exercises included in this section address loud voice production in different ways. Two exercises, Behrman's *Calling the Text* and Phyland's *"Cooee" (The Aussie Bushman's Call),* use calls with different vowel sequences containing rapid changes in pitch and loudness, to achieve the breath support and vocal tract postures that facilitate an easily produced loud voice. Chan's *The Power of the Amplifier* guides the client in maintaining resonant voice production while using a microphone. Klimek's *Using Twang* teaches loudness using a vocal quality often referred to as "bright" or even "piercing" through manipulation of the shape of the vocal tract, particularly the supraglottis and velopharyngeal port. Ostrowski's *Vocal Intensity Play* incorporates singing voice techniques, promoting smooth transitions between soft and loud voice to help the client maintain appropriate breath use and vocal tract resonance in louder voice production. For most clients, these exercises, particularly *Calling the Text, "Cooee" (The Aussie Bushman's Call)*, and *The Power of the Amplifier*, are best used only after the client has achieved the prerequisite skills of good speech-breathing support and resonant voice. And therapists will find some of these exercises, particularly *Using Twang* and *Vocal Intensity Play*, excellent tasks to use with clients working on other goals, such as exploration of pitch or release of hyperfunction.

It may be helpful for therapists to discuss with their clients how and where to practice these exercises between therapy sessions. Some clients may find it difficult to generate a loud voice by themselves, perhaps in a quiet environment, without a therapist to coach them. Others may feel hesitant to produce loud voice within earshot of friends or neighbors. Possible solutions include playing the radio or TV moderately loudly, which can help to mask the client's loud voice and, at the same time, help the client to gauge whether the voice production is sufficiently loud. For clients who live near traffic noise, practicing by an open window may be a possibility. And practicing in the car with the radio playing can offer a good opportunity for uninhibited loud voice use.

When your therapy sessions target healthy and efficient loud voice production, we encourage you to consider exercises from other sections in this book, many of which can be explored using louder voice after the client has achieved success at a softer conversational level.

Calling the Text

Alison Behrman

Purpose

■ To achieve loud voice production in an easy and healthy manner.

Origin

This exercise was inspired by Arthur Lessac's famous "call" (Lessac, 1960). He used the term *call* to refer to a sound produced in the upper two-thirds of the vocal range, using an open oropharyngeal space, to yield a loud, rich sound produced with little effort. I observed a variation of this exercise developed by Jeanie LoVetri, a singing teacher in New York City. I adapted Jeanie's exercise for the speaking voice, initially for a client who works on a financial trading floor. Subsequently, I found the exercise helpful for many clients who needed to talk loudly from time to time.

Overview

In this exercise, a "call" is produced at the beginning of a phrase to establish a resonant, loud voice. The key to producing a loud voice in an easy and healthy manner lies in strong abdominal breath control and lack of hyperfunction in the vocal tract. When produced accurately, the call is achieved with a sensation of openness and resonant forward sound (sensation of ease and forward vibration). The call is blended into each phrase, starting with words and short phrases that are designed to facilitate resonant voice production, and then progressing to more complex sentences and spontaneous speech. The client is encouraged to capture the sensation of the call (open throat, good breath support) and carry it through to the spoken text.

Note: I introduce this exercise later in the therapy process, after the client has established good speech-breathing habits, resonant voice production, and appropriate articulatory movement. This exercise is contraindicated for clients with phonotrauma.

The Exercise

1. Practice the call "yellooo!" at a comfortably loud level (the word *yellow* with the final vowel prolonged). Pretend you are

> Other calls that can be useful to facilitate easy and healthy loud voice production include the call used on a pig farm ("sooeee"), the howls of a dog or wolf (or werewolf, if you prefer), and the siren of emergency vehicles.

Optional Negative Practice. Sometimes it can be helpful to engage the client in "negative practice." After the client has achieved success with the call and phrases, ask the client to say a few of the same phrases without the call "the old way," focusing the energy in the throat. Ask the client to compare the sensations and sound of the voice when produced the "old" and "new" ways.

Optional Pitch Range Extension. After the client has achieved success using the call to achieve a comfortably loud voice, encourage the client to focus now on maintaining a wide range of pitches (slightly exaggerated) throughout the call and subsequent phrases. Next, slowly fade the call and maintain the exaggerated pitch range throughout the phrases. And, finally, moderate the exaggerated pitch so that the phrases are produced with an appropriately wide pitch range.

calling out into a canyon to generate an echo. A low, open breath should precede the call. The call is produced with a low and relaxed jaw. The /l/ consonant should be produced with the tongue tip quite far in the front of the mouth. And finally, the /o/ is produced with a low jaw position and gently rounded lips. The pitch may glide downward a bit but don't let it drop too low. It is important that the call be mastered before progressing on to the next step.

2. Produce the call "yellooo" and allow it to blend into each of the following words, as in yelloooWon!:

   Wonderful!

   We won!

   Why not!

   Welcome everyone!

Throughout each of the words following the call, maintain a sense of energy at the front of the mouth. Even as the pitch descends a bit at the end of the phrase, do not allow the energy to fall off or stop the breath before the end of the phrase.

3. Produce the call "yellooo" with other phrases and sentences. Strive to maintain energy in the lips and tongue tip throughout the phrase.

4. Repeat Steps 2 and 3, but this time just "think" the call, recalling the sensation and allowing time to breathe, but not actually producing the call out loud.

'Cooee' (The Aussie Bushman's Call)

Debbie Phyland

Purposes

To facilitate:

- Forward oral resonance.
- Increased control of pitch variation and widened pitch range through improved speech-breathing support.
- Loud voice production in an easy and healthy manner.

Origin

In Australia, a well-known call is used, when one is out in the bush, to register distress or seek help. The call is meant to be reserved for emergencies but it is frequently used playfully in a big reverberating space. It is thought to be adapted from the indigenous people, who in turn had probably imitated the call of the "cooee bird," or koel (*Eudynamys scolopacea*). Many voice therapists in Australia have found this bush call to be quite useful as "vocal play" in therapy for promoting improved resonance and optimizing control of loudness and pitch changes.

Overview

The call is produced with an emphasis on forward oral resonance and good speech-breathing support. Dynamic and exaggerated use of the lower thoracic and abdominal muscles is used for a "diaphragm kick" to achieve the rapid upward siren in the second syllable of the call. The result is efficient laryngeal valving and a concentration of acoustic energy in the supraglottal vocal tract.

The Exercise

1. Practice the call "cooee." The /ku/ part of the call begins at a comfortable speaking pitch and is prolonged at that pitch for approximately 3 seconds with strong forward oral resonance. Then siren up quickly on the /wi/, finishing on a short, high note. Use a rapid contraction of the abdominal muscles (a quick "diaphragm kick") as you siren upward in pitch. The call should be produced at a comfortably loud level, and it should be smoothly continuous throughout, without any interruptions in voicing or breath flow. Practice the call 5 to 10 times without strain.

2. After you achieve consistent success in producing the call appropriately, practice using it before a variety of utterances spoken at a moderately loud level while using forward resonance and exaggerated breath control.

The Power of the Amplifier

Karen M. K. Chan

Purposes

- To vary loudness appropriately while using a microphone.
- To maintain appropriate resonance while using a microphone.

Origin

This exercise was inspired by the Lessac-Madsen Resonant Voice Therapy (LMRVT) program, in which generalization of the resonant voice to daily life is trained in different contexts, such as talking on the telephone or with background noise. Many of my clients report that their voice sounds different and tires easily when using a microphone. This exercise addresses that concern.

Overview

This exercise is designed for clients who are nearing the end of therapy and who could benefit from using a microphone at work (such as teachers and others who speak to large groups). It is assumed that the client can produce resonant voice at sentence level or above. This exercise will train the patients to listen to their voice with and without the microphone and how to use the microphone appropriately.

Note: If possible, practice in a room that has acoustics similar to the client's actual work environment. For example, if the client typically speaks against background noise, have the client practice with a radio playing. Ask the client to bring work materials to the therapy sessions, such as a lesson plan or business products, to practice an actual presentation.

The Exercise

1. Stand in the middle of the room and pretend that you are at work. Say a few sentences as you normally would at work.
2. Evaluate how well your voice seemed to carry across the room. Did the loudness level seem to be sufficient for your typical work environment?

> The therapist may want to introduce different types of microphones and amplification systems and work with the client to determine the optimal system. Instruct the client to hold the microphone lightly in one hand, with its head just below the lips and angled directly at the mouth. Make sure that the client is not speaking into the side of the microphone head.

The therapist can guide the client to monitor a variety of parameters while using the microphone, such as speaking rate, pitch, resonance, mouth-to-microphone distance, and loudness level. During practice, the client can monitor one parameter for a few sentences, then move on to the next parameter for the next set of sentences, and so on.

After the client has achieved some success maintaining a resonant voice with the microphone, have the client begin to speak with the amplifier turned off but holding the microphone. When the client can project the voice well with appropriate resonance, turn the amplifier on and off periodically to ensure that the client does not alter vocal resonance with the amplifier turned on.

3. Repeat Step 1 using a microphone and amplifier. Do not speak down to the microphone. Your head should remain level and you should continue to look out at your "audience." Imagine that you are sending your voice out across the room even though you are speaking directly into the microphone. Maintain frontal/oral resonance while using the microphone. Compare the resonance of your voice when speaking with and without the microphone.

4. When you can maintain appropriate resonance during short sentence production while using the microphone, progress to longer utterances. Continue to simulate real work speaking situations.

Vocal Intensity Play

Rosemary Ostrowski

Purposes

To facilitate:

- More efficient production of loud voice by maximizing vocal tract filter function.
- An increase in pitch and loudness ranges (vocal flexibility).
- Use of sensory awareness of facial vibrations for controlling resonance.

Origin

These exercises are based on Directed Energy Voice Technique (DEVT), developed by William Riley, a singing voice specialist with whom I had the good fortune to train and work for many years. Singers are expected to produce a pleasant yet energetic sound while maintaining healthy vocal folds throughout frequent performances. DEVT guides the singer to use the vocal tract as an efficient filter of the voice source signal, thus avoiding use of forceful "misdirected" energy. It is hypothesized that efficient filtering allows the singer to avoid the potentially phonotraumatic vocal behaviors of excessive subglottal pressure and laryngeal muscle constriction, particularly when using a loud voice. This principle should hold true for the speaking voice as well. Vocal Intensity Play, my adaptation of DEVT for the speaking voice, is based on the premise that use of a loud speaking voice can be achieved in a healthy manner by maximizing the filter function of the vocal tract.

Overview

Vocal Intensity Play uses the **messa di voce**, a classical operatic training technique involving **crescendo-diminuendo**, or soft-to-loud-to-soft production. The intensity shifts are designed to promote a balance among the intrinsic muscles of the larynx with changing lung pressures. Use of a breathy vocal quality is avoided, because the excessive airflow associated with breathiness limits the effectiveness of the vocal tract to maintain vocal energy. The word "play" was chosen because it allows the speaker to explore vocal boundaries by shifting vocal intensity. Playing with the voice may promote greater vocal flexibility, providing more vocal choices to

> The client does not have to be a singer to benefit from these exercises, but the client should be able to match pitches with relative accuracy and ease. The therapist does not need to be a singer, but should have basic music theory knowledge and access to a keyboard.

meet the varied communicative needs of the speaker, thereby promoting vocal health.

Note: The exercises utilize approximately 13 semitones (one octave) of the speaking range of the client. The starting note can be adjusted for individual clients and it is not necessary to use the entire octave, particularly in the early stages of practice.

The Exercises

Guide the client to focus on the sensation of energy or buzz in the front of the face or on the hard palate, rather than focusing on the sound of the voice. Recommend that the client audio record the therapy session to use as guidance during home practice.

The client may perform the exercises sitting or standing, as long as the posture allows a low breath. In either case, the sternum should be comfortably high, rib cage lifted, shoulders back and down with the scapulae mildly retracted. If the client is standing, the knees should be unlocked. No strain or discomfort should be experienced. The jaw should remain relaxed and "unhinged" with the lips slightly protruded to facilitate maximum oral resonance. A sensation of vibration or energy should be experienced in the front of the face or the hard palate during production of the exercises. Alternatively, a sensation of *absence* of tension in the throat is a good indication that the sound has been well directed.

The exercises should be repeated two to three times up and down the octave for approximately 5 minutes. The exercise can be performed two to three times daily and can be adjusted to the needs of the client. The goal is to feel the vibrations on the bones of the face.

1. Sliding Thirds

   In a speechlike manner, say /wɑː u/ sliding up and down a major third. The first syllable /wɑ/ should be a bright sound (loud) on the onset. The second syllable /u/ should be a dark sound (soft). The tone should be soft but not breathy. Good speech-breathing support should be maintained, using a low breath. However, not much air is needed to produce the slide up and down, so avoid overbreathing. Try to feel the vibration on the bones of the face. The slide should be produced in a light manner and the tones should be easy and free of strain.

2. Ji-Je-Jo Descending Scale

Say each syllable of /ji je jo/ with a quick intensity shift (loud to soft) following by a descending five-tone scale on /o/. Let your tongue move forward and high for the /j/. The sides of the tongue should touch the top molars and the tip should be down behind the bottom teeth. The tongue position will compress the air as it courses through the mouth, causing a buzz on the hard palate and producing an intense sound. Tone production should be easy. Begin the exercise on a pitch that is five tones up from the lowest pitch to accommodate the descending scale.

2A Female (range A3-A4)

Continue exercise up to A4 (440Hz)

2B Male (range A2-A3)

Continue exercise up to A3 (220Hz)

Using Twang

Mary McDonald Klimek

Purposes

To increase:

- Clarity of the voice.
- Ease of voice production.
- Loudness level without strain or effort.

Origin

I used twang voice quality back in 1979 to 1980 when I studied singing with Adele Addison at the Aspen Music School and in New York City. Many singing voice teachers employ twang, although it can be referred to by different names. My use of twang in the voice therapy clinic has been informed by my work in Estill Voice Training with Jo Estill and Kimberly Steinhauer, Ph.D.

Overview

Use of twang quality can be helpful in cases of both hypo- and hyperfunctional voice production to yield a clearer and louder voice produced with greater ease and less vocal strain. This exercise teaches the client to achieve twang voice quality through imitation of a number of commonly known voices of actors, cartoon characters, and even animal sounds. A slight nasal quality combined with a playful and somewhat silly approach is used to minimize potential hyperfunction while facilitating the twang.

The point of this exercise is not to have the client habituate a consistent twang quality to be used routinely in conversational voice (although several regional accents in the United States do feature twang). Rather, the therapeutic intent is to facilitate a slight (*lingering*) twang quality that may facilitate more efficient and easier voice production. Where I, myself, might *consciously* add twang (or, more likely subtract it, as my voice can err on the "bright" side), when I work with dysphonic voices I find that simply "priming" the voice with a good bit of twang is sufficient to alter the production that follows.

Note: The following are assumed:

- The therapist understands the difference between epilaryngeal narrowing and velopharyngeal port opening.
- The client has demonstrated a willingness to be playful.

Editors' Note: What is *twang*? Many people would respond with "nasal," as in "the nasal twang of a New Yorker" or "that nasal twang in country music." In fact, some twang has a nasal quality and some twang does not, as differentiated by an open or closed velopharyngeal port. One hears the twang quality in a classic witch's cackle or schoolyard "nyae-nyae" taunt.

Acoustically, the frequency characteristics of twang correspond to that of the singer's formant, with a power spectrum peak in the region between 2000 and 4000 Hz. The high frequency energy is often described as a very "bright" or even "piercing" sound that has a strong "ring." Aesthetically, twang does not appeal to everyone, and yet it produces a singing voice that is more easily heard over an orchestra without amplification, and a speaking voice that can be heard above the din of a noisy room.

Biomechanically, it is believed that twang is achieved with a narrowed epilaryngeal space or aryepiglottic sphincter (AES). The key, however, is to achieve anteroposterior narrowing of the upper epilarynx while avoiding mediolateral compression of the supraglottis at the level of the false vocal folds. Adding a slight nasal quality by opening the the velopharyngeal port can facilitate the target vocal tract posture.

The Exercise

1. Finding happy twang

Try any or all of the following prompts to establish a twang training gesture:

- The childhood taunt,
  "nyae   nyae   nyae   nyae   nyae"
              nyae
- Cackling like a witch, "yeh-heh-heh!"
- Calling "Patrick!" like Sponge Bob Squarepants
- "Baaaaa"-*ing* like a sheep
- "Neigh"-*ing* like a horse
- "Nyuk-nyuk-nyuk"-*ing* like The Three Stooges
- "MBeep-beep" like Road-Runner
- "Oh, Mr. Sheffield!" like The Nanny
- (Add your own)

Note that twang vocal quality is not achieved by simply making the voice louder, which can place you at risk for vocal strain. Instead, the sound you produce should be very bright, but *fun* to listen to and *fun* to produce. The kinesthetic sensations associated with happy twang may be perceived as "forward" and in the nose or imaginary muzzle, or behind and below the base of the tongue.

2. Putting twang to work

Here are a few suggestions:

Prime your voice with twang by inserting your happiest twang training gesture before:

- Speaking a word, phrase, or sentence
- Reading a paragraph
- Reciting a nursery rhyme, psalm, the Pledge of Allegiance

You can also use a twang "template" in common daily functional phrases (such as "Hi! How are you? Or "Thank you very much") or in a "carrier phrase" by filling in the blanks with numbers, days, months, ice cream flavors, or objects in the room, for example. Twang your happiest training gesture in the pitch and stress contour and rhythm of the phrase prior to speaking it.

Fade the use of the twang training gesture as clarity and ease are consistently achieved

---

Avoiding Unhappy Twang.

If your voice sounds shrill and could make a listener uncomfortable, you are most likely using false vocal fold constriction. (We might say you have a cork stuck in your throat.)

The kinesthetic sensations associated with unhappy twang are:

An itch, tickle, or scratch in the laryngeal area (*not* "most comfortable vocal effort")

A strangling blockage in the laryngeal area

Helpful Hints:

I usually give my clients (and myself) "3 Strikes"—if successive approximation toward a happier twang is just not happening, we step away and regroup.

Nasalizing will help, somewhat. Have the client exhale a puff of breath through the nose prior to each vocalization.

Have the client exhale to resting expiratory level before twanging to reduce the relaxation pressure beneath the voice.

To further reduce the risk of false vocal fold constriction during twang production, instruct the client to make the twang training gestures softly, with "small" bright cartoon character voices, such as *happy* witches.

Keeping the tongue high and the space in the mouth "small" will also help. I often instruct patients to say the "nyae's" or "nyuk's" as if they were scraping peanut butter off the roof of their mouths—the way dogs do, scraping *forward*.

Hand signals sometimes help. Generally, I mime the anteroposterior narrowing just in front of my neck. Letting the hands "make" the sound adds another layer of silliness and play, further reducing the risk of false vocal fold constriction.

Chapter 9

FACILITATING EFFICIENT VOCAL FOLD CLOSURE

Efficiency of vocal fold vibration is a goal that infuses all of our therapy approaches, but in this chapter we address, in particular, the problem of insufficient vocal fold closure. In general, many of us are hesitant to promote effortful closure that could lead to excessive muscle contractions, for then we have the problem of vocal hyperfunction. Instead, our goal is to achieve good vocal fold closure efficiently, through maximal coordination between the airflow and the tension settings of the vocal folds. In this way, we seek to achieve the best closure that our clients can produce easily and that generates a clear voice.

Eight exercises are included in this section. Stemple's *Vocal Function Exercises* (VFEs) are well known to many in the voice therapy community. VFEs include warm-up, stretching, contracting, and low impact adductory power tasks to help strengthen the laryngeal muscles and improve vocal fold adduction.

Both Carroll's *Vocal Fry to Modal* and Medrado's *Vocal Fry* take advantage of the differences in vocal fold tension across different speaking registers to help the client achieve increased control of vocal fold vibration and improved glottal closure. Vocal fry is achieved with greater laxness of the vocal folds, and increased contact of the tissue. As the client shifts from vocal fry to modal register, the goal is to maintain some of the elements of the lower register to heighten closure. Haxer's *Hypofunctional Dysphonia* uses triggers such as a cough or throat-clear, to facilitate more complete closure. Other facilitative techniques, including use of chanting and semioccluded vocal tract, are then linked to the trigger to further shape the phonation. Miller's *Sharp Onset* uses modified hard onsets in text loaded with initial vowels, to achieve improved closure. In *Up and Down Staccato*, Miller again uses a modification of hard glottal attacks, here coordinated with changes in pitch, to facilitate improved vocal fold closure. Ziegler and Hapner's *Phonation Resistance Training Exercise (PhoRTE) Therapy* targets muscular strength and endurance in clients with age-related changes to the vocal folds that often result in persistent glottal gap during phonation. And Pinho's

Retention of Spaghetti focuses on breath control, using a sipping maneuver, to increase closure.

In addition to the exercises in this section, we are confident that you will find other exercises throughout this book that are beneficial for your clients with impaired vocal fold closure. Often, improving speech-breathing support, reducing supraglottal vocal tract hyperfunction through attention to articulation, and achieving forward resonance, can serve to improve the efficiency and clarity of the voice, even in the presence of imperfect vocal fold closure.

Vocal Function Exercises

Joseph C. Stemple

Purposes

Vocal Function Exercises represent a series of systematic exercises designed:

- To strengthen and balance the laryngeal musculature
- To improve vocal fold adduction
- To coordinate the subsystems of voice production: respiration, phonation, and resonance.

Origin

A series of laryngeal muscle exercises was first described by Briess (1957, 1959). He suggested that there is a direct relationship between the condition of the laryngeal musculature and the quality of voice, and that, for the voice to be most effective, the intrinsic muscles of the larynx must be in a dynamic equilibrium. I modified and expanded these exercises into Vocal Function Exercises (VFE) (Stemple, 1984).

Overview

The program begins by describing the vocal problem to the client, using illustrations as needed, or the client's own stroboscopic evaluation video. The client is then taught a series of four specific vocal exercises, completed two times each, two times per day, preferably morning and evening. Commonly, this exercise program will be performed for 6 to 8 weeks; however, this time period may vary. The first exercise in the series is considered a vocal warm-up that helps to engage the laryngeal system. The second exercise promotes stretching of the vocal folds by requiring the individual to slowly glide in an ascending manner through the pitch range. The third exercise promotes contraction of the vocal folds by requiring the individual to slowly glide in a descending manner through the pitch range. The fourth exercise serves as a low-impact adductory strengthening, or "power exercise," and requires the individual to sustain five sequential musical notes for as long as possible. All four exercises in the program are produced with an engaged laryngeal muscle system and a front tone focus that partially occludes the vocal tract. The exercises are simple to teach and, when presented

For a more thorough description of vocal function exercises, their theoretical basis, and specific steps, see *Clinical Voice Pathology: Theory and Management* (4th ed.) (Stemple, Glaze, & Klaben, 2009).

appropriately, seem reasonable to clients. It has been my experience that many clients are enthusiastic about a concrete program, similar in concept to physical therapy, during which they may chart the progress of their return to vocal efficiency. The exercises are equally effective with vocal hyperfunction or hypofunction. All exercises are produced as softly as possible, but not breathy.

Vocal Function Exercise Practice Record   **TARGET: _____ seconds**

Week 1			1st Day	2nd	3rd	4th	5th	6th	7th
		DATE							
AM	1	**"Eee"** *Sustain the vowel "ee" for as long as you can. Placement should be extremely forward, almost but not quite nasal. Do this as soft as possible, but not breathy. Engage the voice. This is a warm-up. Time this exercise. Record times for 2 attempts below.*							
			/	/	/	/	/	/	/
	2	**Glide from your lowest note to your highest on "knoll."** *You may also choose to use "woo" or "whoops." Check off 2 attempts at this exercise, but you do not need to time or measure the pitch. The goal is no voice breaks, and buzzing in the lips.*							
			☐☐	☐☐	☐☐	☐☐	☐☐	☐☐	☐☐
	3	**Glide from a comfortable high pitch to your lowest pitch on "knoll."** *You may also choose to use "woo" or "whoops." Check off 2 attempts at this exercise, but you do not need to time or measure the pitch. The goal is no voice breaks, and buzzing in the lips.*							
			☐☐	☐☐	☐☐	☐☐	☐☐	☐☐	☐☐
	4	**Sustain the following 5 ascending pitches** *for as long as possible on the sound "ooooo." This should also feel buzzy in the lips. If you place a finger in front of your mouth you feel a narrow stream of air for as long as you voice.*							
		Pitch 1	/	/	/	/	/	/	/
		Pitch 2	/	/	/	/	/	/	/
		Pitch 3	/	/	/	/	/	/	/
		Pitch 4	/	/	/	/	/	/	/
		Pitch 5	/	/	/	/	/	/	/
PM	1	"Eee"	/	/	/	/	/	/	/
	2	Up glide	☐☐	☐☐	☐☐	☐☐	☐☐	☐☐	☐☐
	3	Low glide	☐☐	☐☐	☐☐	☐☐	☐☐	☐☐	☐☐
	4	Pitch 1	/	/	/	/	/	/	/
		Pitch 2	/	/	/	/	/	/	/
		Pitch 3	/	/	/	/	/	/	/
		Pitch 4	/	/	/	/	/	/	/
		Pitch 5	/	/	/	/	/	/	/

The Exercise

1. Warm-Up: Sustain the /i/ vowel for as long as possible on a musical note (F) above middle (C) for females and boys, and (F) below middle (C) for males. The notes may be modified up or down to fit individual needs, but seldom by more than two notes in either direction. If you have airflow measurement instrumentation available, your goal is to reach 80 to 100 mL/second. For example, if the flow volume is 40,000 mL, then the goal is 40 to 45 seconds. If instrumentation is not available, your goal is to sustain the /i/ for as long as you are able to sustain an /s/. Placement of the tone should be in an extreme forward focus, almost, but not quite, nasal.

2. Stretching: Glide from your lowest note to your highest note on the word "Knoll" (sustaining the "l"). Make sure to keep your lips rounded. You should feel vibration in your lips. Your goal is to produce the glide without any voice breaks. If you do experience a voice break (particularly in the transition between low and high registers), try to continue the glide without hesitation. If voice breaks occur or phonation stops toward the top of your range, the glide may be continued without voice, as the vocal folds will continue to stretch.

3. Contraction: Glide from a comfortable high note to your lowest note on the word "Knoll" (sustaining the "l" sound). As you glide, try to feel a half-yawn in your throat. Again, your goal is to produce the glide without voice breaks and to feel vibration in the lips.

4. Low Impact Adductory Power: Sustain the musical notes (C-D-E-F-G) for as long as possible on the word "old" without the "d" (again, sustaining the "l" sound). Use middle C for females and boys, and an octave below middle C for males. The goal remains the same, to produce the glide without voice breaks and to feel vibration in the lips.

> In Stretching (Step 2), the glide requires the use of all laryngeal muscles. It stretches the vocal folds and encourages a systematic, slow engagement of the cricothyroid muscles, thereby improving muscular control and flexibility. The word "knoll" encourages an expanded open pharynx, as well as a forward placement of the tone and the rounded, almost closed lips occlude the vocal tract. Pharyngeal and lip posture is similar to that of an inverted megaphone. As an option, the client may also use a lip trill, tongue trill, or the word "whoop" or "molm."
>
> In Contraction (Step 3), by keeping the pharynx open and focusing the sympathetic vibration at the lips, the downward glide encourages a slow, systematic engagement of the thyroarytenoid muscles without the presence of a back-focused growl. In fact, no growl is permitted. As an option, you may also use a lip trill, tongue trill, or the word "boom." The shape of the pharynx to the lips is likened to an inverted megaphone.

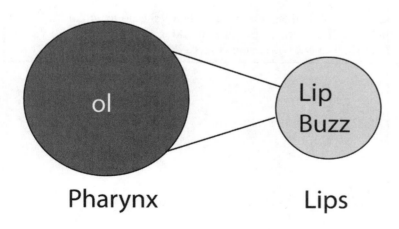

Pharynx   Lips

Therapy Notes. The quality of the sustained tones is also monitored for voice breaks, wavering, and breathiness. Quality improves as times increase and closure improves, and pathologies begin to resolve. All exercises are done softly, but engaged, with a forward tone that lacks tension. In addition, attention is paid to the glottal onset of the tone. The client is asked to breathe in deeply with attention paid to the following sequence: training abdominal breathing, shaping the vowel, and then initiating the exercise gesture without a forceful glottal attack or an aspirate breathy attack. It is explained to the client that maximum phonation times increase as the efficiency of the vocal fold vibration improves. Times do not increase with improved lung capacity. The musical notes are matched to the notes produced by an inexpensive pitch pipe, keyboard, or a digital keyboard available for free download on a computer or smartphone, such as http://www.virtualpiano.com/ Alternatively, the CD that accompanies this book contains a live voice recording. Many clients find the audio-recorded voice easier to match. Finally, clients are given a chart on which to mark the timing of their sustained tones; a means of plotting progress. Estimated time of completion for the program is 6 to 8 weeks, but may vary with age and ability.

Maintenance. When the client has reached the predetermined therapy goal, and the voice quality and other vocal symptoms have improved, then a tapering maintenance program is recommended. Although some of the professional voice users choose to remain in peak vocal condition and continue daily VFEs, many patients desire to taper the VFE program. The following systematic taper is recommended:

- Full program 2 times each, 2 times per day
- Full program 2 times each, 1 time per day (morning)
- Full program 1 time each, 1 time per day (morning)
- Exercise #4, 2 times each, 1 time per day (morning)
- Exercise #4, 1 time each, 1 time per day (morning)
- Exercise #4, 1 time each, 3 times per week (morning)
- Exercise #4, 1 time each, 1 time per week (morning)

Each taper should last one week. Clients should maintain 85% of their peak time, otherwise they should move up one step in the taper until the 85% criterion is met.

Vocal Fry to Modal

Linda M. Carroll

Purpose

■ To increase control of vocal fold vibration in the presence of a mass lesion such as a polyp.

Origin

When I was a teenager growing up in Maine, and learning how to drive, my father taught me how to control skidding on an icy roadway by pulling myself out of the skid. I think of the task of stabilizing the asymmetry of vocal fold vibration in the presence of a mass lesion such as a polyp, as analogous to controlling a skid.

I designed this exercise with the hypothesis that polyps cause aperiodicity of vocal fold vibration, and that manipulation of the vocal folds with the added mass of the polyp is difficult. Vocal fry is a sustained, aperiodic mode of phonation. Changing from highly aperiodic phonation (vocal fry) on a neutral low vowel /ɑ/ and sliding up to a modal /u/ allows the client to learn how to manipulate vocal fold mass and achieve greater periodicity of vocal fold vibration.

Overview

This exercise can be useful for both singers and nonsingers. The therapist and client, without musical backgrounds, need only to be able to move from vocal fry to a modal pitch, and move around in the modal register with short vowel glides. The therapist begins the exercise by defining and demonstrating vocal fry. The exercise is practiced only in midrange, with limited extension upward in succeeding trials.

The Exercise

1. Sustain /ɑ/ in the fry register for two or three seconds. Then slide from fry up into /u/ in modal register. Sustain the /u/ for a second, and then slide down the scale like a sigh. Be sure to maintain modal register through the downward slide.
2. Repeat the exercise several times, allowing the slide up from fry into /u/ to go higher in the pitch range.

Vocal Fry Associated with High-Pitched Blow Sound

Reny Medrado

Purpose

■ To improve phonatory glottal closure in clients with breathy voices.

Origin

This exercise builds on the use of vocal fry as a therapeutic technique. I learned about the high-pitched blow sound from my professor, Dr. Mara Behlau. After working with these two techniques separately, I started to combine them, and found that using the combination worked especially well with clients who presented with a soft, breathy voice.

Overview

The exercise must be done with complete relaxation of the vocal mechanism, and with steady breath support. The therapist must be able to model the two vocal productions without strain.

The Exercise

1. Produce vocal fry on the vowel /a/ for a few seconds, with a continuous creaky sound.
2. Now, purse your lips in a blow position, and blow out some air.
3. Take another breath, and as you blow out the air, add a high-pitched sound, using either /u/ or /i/.
4. When you can produce both vocal fry and a high-pitched blow sound, alternate: first the fry, then the blow sound, in a connected fashion for at least seven consecutive repetitions.
5. After you are comfortable alternating the fry and the high pitch, practice extending the high pitch into other vowels and then phrases.

Hypofunctional Dysphonia

Marc Haxer

Purpose

- To facilitate improved coordination of breathing and phonation in clients with hypofunctional dysphonias.

Origin

I was introduced to this exercise a number of years ago by my friend and colleague, Jan Lewin, Ph.D. It was her modifications of a protocol that she presented some years earlier on functional dysphonias given by another friend and colleague, Robert E. ("Ed") Stone, Ph.D.

Overview

This exercise begins with a trigger, such as a cough or throat-clear. The voicing produced with the trigger is then shaped into balanced voice production.

Note: Before the exercise is begun, the therapist should explain to the client the nature of his or her voice problem. No time frame is set for working through the tasks. Building and maintaining client confidence is crucial to successful outcome.

Note: Steps that are preceded by an asterisk (*) can be performed simultaneously by the therapist and the client, should that be helpful in certain cases. However, the therapist should gradually stop accompanying the client.

The Exercise

1. Relax your shoulders, using a mirror for visual feedback.
2. Establish low (abdominal) breathing, using a volitional outward movement of the abdomen during inhalation and an inward movement during exhalation ("push out/pull in"). Maintain an open mouth and relaxed throat, focusing on a relaxed exhalation with no sound.
3. *Initiate use of a phonatory trigger, such as a cough, throat-clear, gargle, high-pitched squeak, or "meow."

4. *Once voicing can be produced consistently during repetition of the triggers, increase the consistency and duration of the phonation.

5. *Transition smoothly without pausing from the trigger into a pitch glide /u/ (high to low and then low to high).

6. *Now produce the glide and sustain the sound at a comfortable pitch in the middle of your range.

7. Transition from the glide and sustained sound to a hum.

8. *Slowly alternate between the closed (very resonant) hum and the open and relaxed sigh, as in /mːɑ mːɑː/ in a chant (monotonic). Another sound combination you might try is /ijɑːjɑː/.

9. *Produce the hum and smoothly transition into rote speech tasks in a monotonic chant (legato- or linking-style of speech on a single pitch), such as

   "mmmmmone-two-three-four-five"

   "mmmmMonday-Tuesday-Wednesday-Thursday-Friday"

10. *Drop the hum and instead, use a hand gesture as a visual cue to maintain the chant, increasing the speed as needed to achieve normal rate.

11. Repeat the rote speech tasks maintaining the legato- or linking-style of speaking but instead of monotone, use a natural pitch contour.

12. Continue with more complex speech material.

Sharp Onset Vowel Sentences

Susan Miller

Purpose

■ To improve glottal closure for phonation.

Origin

Voice therapy for individuals with paretic vocal folds or presbylaryngis aims to improve glottal closure while developing abdominal support for breathing, intrinsic muscle strength, and laryngeal adductory and abductory agility. Historically, effortful closure of the glottis achieved by forced adduction exercises were taught to help the uninvolved vocal fold cross over the midline to achieve closure with the paralyzed vocal fold during phonation (Boies, Hilger, & Priest, 1964; Froeschels, Kastein, & Weiss, 1955; Gleason, 1928). As forceful closure frequently creates supraglottic hyperfunction, forceful adduction exercises have been replaced by hard glottal attack exercises to accomplish similar goals (Heuer et al., 1997; Stemple, Lee, et al., 1994; Yamaguchi, Yotsukura, Sata, et al., 1993).

Note: Frequent use of hard glottal attacks may promote phonotrauma in cases where vocal fold contact is achieved and, therefore, this exercise should be used with caution.

Overview

The following exercise is meant to initiate breath support quickly while improving glottal adduction within sentences loaded with vowel-initiated words. It is hypothesized that clients with vocal fold paresis and presbylaryngis can improve vocal fold adduction by performing this exercise twice daily. Most likely, the vowel onsets will be breathy and rough at the beginning but the sound should become less breathy and sharper in onset over time.

Note: Therapists can supplement the words and sentences provided as examples with their own materials. Clients should be cautioned against overpracticing the material to avoid hyperfunctional vocal behaviors.

The Exercise

1. Say each of the following vowels with a forceful effort (sharp onset) at a comfortable pitch: /e/ /i/ /ɑɪ/ /o/ /u/.

2. Say the following words with sharp onsets: Amy, Even, Ice, Own, Umbrella.

3. Use sharp onsets in the following sentences laden with vowel-initiated words. Be sure to produce the beginning of each word sharply. Your sentences will not sound smooth and natural. They will be very abrupt and staccato-sounding. The goal is to close your vocal folds briskly. The underlined vowels are to be produced sharply.

Ellen offered eight examples of arithmetic exercises.

I ordered an apple, artichoke, and egg omelet.

Every American enjoys attending Italian Operas.

Olive introduced Amy to Uncle Ed energetically.

I attended an auction in October in Upper Iceland.

4. Practice saying these five (or similar) sentences one time each in the morning and in the evening for four weeks. Do not say them more than one time each or more than five sentences during one practice session. Over time, as you achieve success with better vocal fold closure, decrease the frequency of the practice.

Up and Down Staccato

Susan Miller

Purpose

■ To improve glottal closure for phonation.

Origin

Most singers engage in a warm-up routine prior to singing, which usually consists of pitch glides and **arpeggios**. These exercises are meant to initiate breath support quickly while stretching the vocal folds and coordinating intrinsic muscle movements. Clients with vocal fold paresis and presbylaryngis can improve vocal fold adduction by performing daily voice exercises utilizing a modification of Titze's staccato on arpeggio exercise. This exercise originates from a singing exercise, in which hard glottal attacks are modified into staccato vowel onsets for singers during arpeggios to elicit clean and rapid vocal onset while training abductor and adductor muscles simultaneously with tensor muscles (Titze, 2006).

Overview

The exercise consists of **staccato** vowel productions at three different parts of the pitch range. The exercise will aid clients in coordinating breath with vocal fold abduction, adduction, and tensing. Although the sound is dysphonic at first, many clients become pleased with their progress over several weeks. Clients who have a piano may enjoy working up and down the scale with the piano.

Note: Frequent use of hard glottal attacks may promote phonotrauma in cases where vocal fold contact is achieved and, therefore, this exercise should be used with caution.

The Exercise

1. Say each of the following vowels with a forceful effort (sharp onset) at a comfortable pitch: /u/ /i/ /o/.
2. Note whether any vowel feels more comfortable or easy to produce with a sharp onset than the others. Chose one of the vowels and continue to practice attaining a sharp onset on the chosen /u/, /i/, or /o/ sound at a comfortable pitch.

3. Practice producing the chosen vowel in a staccato or sharp onset manner while ascending up the scale as an arpeggio. The numbers 1 and 3 indicate ascending notes on the piano scale for example; mid C-E-C, D-F-D. Go up to as high a pitch as you can without straining. Take a short breath between each series of 1-3-1.

(continue up the scale)

```
                    3
              3   1  1 breath
          3    1  1 breath
      3        1  1 breath
   1  1 breath
```

4. Now practice producing the chosen vowel in a staccato or sharp onset manner while descending from the top of the octave. Maintain the same 1-3-1 relationship of notes in each series, for example, high C-E-C, B-D-B. Descend to as low a pitch as you can, taking a short breath between each series of 1-3-1. Do not worry about being "on key."

```
   3
1  1 breath
      3
   1  1 breath
         3
      1  1 breath
         3
      1  1 breath
```

(continue down the scale)

Practice each ascending arpeggio two times and each descending arpeggio two times during a practice session.

5. Continue the series once in the morning and once in the evening for four weeks. As your voice improves, decrease the series to one practice session per day. If the exercise does not improve the strength of your voice, discontinue the exercise.

Phonation Resistance Training Exercise (PhoRTE) Therapy

Aaron Ziegler and Edie R. Hapner

Purposes

- To improve speech breathing support (increases respiratory muscle activity)
- To improve phonatory glottal closure (increases intrinsic laryngeal muscle activity)
- To raise vocal intensity, with improved vocal quality and increased vocal endurance.

Origin

Individuals with age-related voice changes (presbyphonia) frequently complain of reduced loudness and increased vocal fatigue. The Phonation Resistance Training Exercise (PhoRTE) Therapy program targets changes in muscular strength and endurance of the vocal mechanism that occur with age. This voice therapy program uses progressive resistance training, which has been found in the exercise literature to increase muscular force production and endurance, and improve an individual's ability to carry out daily activities (Peterson, Rhea, Sen, & Gordon, 2010). The PhoRTE Therapy program has its roots in research of Lee Silverman Voice Therapy (Ramig, Countryman, Thompson, & Horii, 1995), exercise physiology, (Garber et al., 2011) and progressive resistance training for age-related changes in limb skeletal muscle (Melov, Tarnopolsky, Beckman, Felkey, & Hubbard, 2007) and motor learning (Schmidt & Lee, 2011).

Overview

PhoRTE Therapy consists of four exercises, the goal of which is to induce changes in muscle structure and function of the vocal mechanism, and reverse the perceived age-related voice changes. The client should perform repetitions of loud voice production (about 8 to 10 repetitions) to the point of muscular fatigue using various speech stimuli. Each session should include two sets of the PhoRTE Therapy exercises with a 1-minute rest between sets. The PhoRTE Therapy program should be completed twice daily. The therapist should reevaluate exercise workload weekly and increase the minimum workload as muscular force and endurance improve.

The workup before commencing the PhoRTE Therapy program:

A. Establish the client's habitual loudness. First, have the client read a standard passage for 3 minutes continuously. Then, analyze the middle 2 minutes of the passage to calculate the client's habitual loudness.

B. Determine the client's vocal intensity range by having the client prolong the vowel /a/ at their minimum and maximum vocal intensity. Compute the vocal intensity range by subtracting the minimum vocal intensity from the maximum vocal intensity. Exercise workload in the PhoRTE Therapy program should start at 50 to 60% of the patient's vocal intensity range (50 to 60% of the maximum intensity). The therapist should increase the vocal intensity by 5 dB increments on a weekly basis until the client reaches the final target of +20 dB SPL above habitual loudness (ideally, 80 to 90 dB SPL). If the client is unable to achieve a 5 dB increase in vocal intensity, then reduce the vocal intensity target to a 3 dB increase.

C. All PhoRTE Therapy voice exercises should be completed in modal register.

The Exercise

Use low abdominal breathing gestures for this exercise. For all four exercises, by the end of therapy, you should strive to achieve a loudness level between 80 and 90 dB, as measured by a sound level meter positioned at a microphone-to-mouth distance of 30 cm. In place of a sound level meter, a number of free sound level meter applications are available for download from the Internet. Note that if you should experience any prolonged discomfort or decline in voice quality from performing the PhoRTE Therapy exercises, stop the exercise and contact your therapist.

1. Sustain the vowel /a/ for as long as you can with a loud, energized voice.
2. Glide from low to high and from high to low on the vowel /a/ over your entire pitch range using a loud, energized voice.
3. Shout functional phrases using a loud and higher-pitched voice, like calling over a fence.
4. Using the same phrases from Step 3, produce a strong, authoritative voice at a low pitch level.

When the formal program has ended, you should perform PhoRTE steps three and four, 3 times per week, but no more than once per day, at your target loudness level.

Retention of Spaghetti

Sílvia Pinho

Purpose

■ To increase vocal fold closure.

Origin

Pushing exercises, associated with Emil Froeschels and others, have traditionally been used for vocal fold paralysis or paresis, and for other conditions involving weak vocal fold closure. Pushing exercises may improve adduction, but may also cause hyperfunction or even mucosal injury, especially if loud phonation is attempted. For several years I thought about the problem of improving vocal fold adduction without injuring the vocal fold mucosa, and finally created the retention of spaghetti exercise. The retention of spaghetti is a variation of pushing, but without voice production.

Overview

The exercise begins by sipping in air with elongation of the vocal tract. The inhalation is followed by firm closure of the vocal folds, yielding an isometric exercise that contrasts muscle contraction with rest in a series of trials. In cases of vocal fold bowing, I ask the client to use pushing techniques, such as pushing against the wall or sitting in a chair and pulling up on the sides. These tasks are performed during the glottal closure part of the exercise. I hypothesize that this exercise develops adductor muscular strength and greater resistance to subglottal pressure, and perhaps an increase in the muscular mass of the vocal folds.

The Exercise

1. Sip in slowly and steadily as if you were sipping in a long strand of spaghetti. Keep sipping until the end of the inspiration. During the sipping, check with your fingers to make sure that your larynx is lowering.
2. At the end of the inhalation, firmly close your vocal folds, as though you were holding your breath. Maintain this closure for one or two seconds.

3. Now open and close your vocal folds 10 times in a row, followed by a minute of easy relaxed breathing. During the opening and closing, although you will inhale small amounts of air with each opening, maintain the low larynx position that you achieved during the sipping activity.

4. Repeat the slow sipping maneuver described in Step 1 above, and then produce one series of 10 repetitions of compression and relaxation in 10 seconds. Follow with a short period of quiet, relaxed breathing to avoid hyperventilation.

Chapter 10

PEDIATRIC VOICE THERAPY

Conducting voice therapy with children presents its own special challenges. Immature understanding of the existence and nature of a voice problem and a sense of "being told what to do" can lead to poor motivation and participation in therapy. Successful pediatric voice therapists draw on principles and methods of speech therapy for language and phonological disorders, to promote the child's active participation, creativity, and independence. As therapists, we know that self-awareness of vocal production, in both adults and children, must be addressed to achieve useful gains in therapy. But many of the parameters of vocal control are highly abstract for a child—pitch, loudness, breath control, and vocal effort, for example—and so we use play and pictures to help make these concepts concrete and real for the child.

Seven exercises are included in this section. Dungan's *Quiet Breath In—Easy Breath Out* provides helpful suggestions for incorporating vocal exercises into a game children will enjoy. Ross-Kugler has contributed four exercises. Two of the exercises are grounded in principles of child empowerment and family therapy, and the child takes an active role in developing strategies to manage vocal behaviors. In *Rewriting the Script*, the therapist helps the child develop play scripts (based on real scenarios in the child's life) that involve yelling. With the help of key family members who participate in the therapy sessions and help in the transfer activities at home, the child devises a healthy and appropriate alternative to yelling in a script with the new behavior. In *Camp Voice*, the child plans for appropriate voice use at a summer camp, and constructs a map with activity areas and the type of voice likely to be used in each area.

With *Voice Drawing* and *Blowing Bubbles*, Ross-Kugler offers ways to help the child understand respiratory flow and vocal prosody in speaking. Along similar lines, Wingate, in *The Owl*, provides a method for making the conceptually challenging parameters of pitch, breath control, and easy onset more easily understood. Finally, in *Birds Talking*, Hersan uses relaxed lip and tongue trills with pitch variation to simulate dialogue for different situations and emotions. Ultimately, the trills become dialogue reflecting these situations and emotions.

Let the seven exercises in this chapter guide you to adapt other exercises throughout this book for your child clients by making them fun and perhaps even a little silly.

Quiet Breath In—Easy Voice Out

Ellen Love Dungan

Purpose

■ To develop an easy voice with a relaxed, open throat.

Origin

I developed these exercises for children who present with voice disorders resulting from vocal habits such as yelling on the playground and extended loud talking. Often, these children, who may have laryngitis or prenodular swelling of the vocal folds, make their voice problems worse by using maladaptive compensatory behaviors in their efforts to achieve vocal fold closure. A goal of therapy is to teach these children how to reduce laryngeal tension to lessen the impact of vocal fold adduction, and to coordinate breath supply with the demands of speech. These goals must be taught in ways that are easy for them to understand and to practice. In developing these exercises, I have found Moya Andrews' loudness scale (2002) to be a useful tool. I have also drawn on phrasing exercises that I use for adults. (See Dungan and Haskell's exercise, *Breathing Awareness* in Chapter 3.)

Overview

I begin the exercises by explaining the concept of "easy voice." An easy voice is a quiet voice. I introduce the loudness scale, with one a very quiet voice and five a very loud voice. An easy voice does not go above three. An easy voice is produced with a relaxed open throat. An easy voice is produced with quiet air in and easy voice out, and with a "quiet h" at the beginning of words that begin with a vowel. The exercises then proceed, over several sessions, through a number of stages of learning.

The Exercises

1. Say the following words and phrases, preceding each one with a quiet /h/. Pause before beginning each new utterance to allow time for a quiet breath in and easy voice out.

/h/I	/h/and	/h/is	/h/as	/h/am	/h/it

    /h/I like pizza.   /h/And I will go.   /h/Is it time?

    /h/As he said.   /h/Am I going?   /h/It is raining.

2. Practice using a quiet breath in and easy voice out in the following tasks. Remember to put a quiet /h/ in front of words that begin with a vowel.

Count from one to 20.

Say the days of the week.

Describe a picture using the phrases "I see a . . ." "And I see a . . ."

Say a nursery rhyme

State three things about an object, for example, the color, the shape, and what it is used for.

Read a story.

Describe how you do something, for example, how do you go to school in the morning?

3. Incorporate practice of a quiet /h/ and easy voice in the following games.

Pick-Up Sticks

Each time you pick up a stick say the appropriate phrase, such as, "I pick up a red stick," using a quiet "h" at the beginning of the phrase.

Memory Game

Each time you turn over a picture card, say an appropriate phrase, such as "I have a (pig)," using a quiet "h" at the beginning. Or make your own memory word cards beginning with a vowel, or short phrase cards with the initial word beginning with a vowel.

Board Games

You can use your favorite board game for practicing your new easy voice. Or you can make your own board game. On poster paper, draw a winding trail that leads from "start" to "finish" with a series of even spaces along the way. Some of the spaces have "chance" written on them. Draw a card with a picture, word, or phrase written on it. Repeat the word or phrase on the card using the new, easy voice. Then, roll the die and move ahead the number of spaces indicated. When you land on a space that says "chance," draw a card. The card may say "Go back two spaces" or it may ask you to use your new easy voice, for example, "Repeat the Pledge of Allegiance using your easy voice and then go ahead two spaces."

Rewriting the "Script"

Leah Ross-Kugler

Purposes

- To minimize habitual yelling or other maladaptive vocal behaviors.
- To increase the child's awareness of phonotraumatic vocal behaviors and empower the child.

Origin

It is often impossible to change the behavior of a "yeller" without including family members or others in the child's immediate environment. I have a strong behavioral orientation, and so I look for safe and nonthreatening ways to modify real-life situations that could be phonotraumatic for the child. Acting or role-playing is an ideal activity. Most children, who are "naturals" at this, become empowered in several ways. Not only do they learn to manage their own vocal behaviors, the behaviors of others may change (for example, less yelling in the home). Parents or caregivers may begin to provide different (and, one hopes, better) models for their children.

The idea of changing the scenario using role-playing originally came from addressing problems in pragmatics with learning-disabled children. Child psychology books, such as Stanley Turecki's *The Difficult Child*, address the idea of discussing planned actions ahead of time.

Overview

During the evaluation, I ask both the child and the parents about any yelling that may occur at home or elsewhere. In a nonjudgmental manner, I will ask: "Who's the loudest person in the house?" and/or "Who's the quietest?" and/or "When does a lot of shouting occur?" It is often the case that all members of the family yell or talk loudly, not just the child. After identifying at-risk situations and working with the child for a few sessions, I may do some script-writing and play-acting with the child. I always try to use humor. Many children think that it is fun when an adult role-plays a "mad child" or an "angry parent."

The exercise given below is an example of the type of play that may emerge. The therapist asks questions and writes down the answers in play form. The child sets the scene and dictates the

Changing the family dialogue has the potential for changing the family dynamic. If a child yells in any context (watching TV, playing on the playground), the therapist needs to help the child find a more desirable behavior that can be substituted for the (less desirable) yelling behavior. Nonverbal substitutes for random yelling can be used by the child. A good example might be a stuffed toy dog with a careful hole created in its belly. A child can pull out all the stuffing when he or she is angry. (Select a toy that can be reused by having the child put the stuffing back inside the toy so that it is ready for the next time it is needed.) Another idea is to give the child a "little angry man," for example, a muscle man toy to carry in a pocket that can "scream" for the child. The child can place his or her fingers on the toy and squeeze, which replaces the scream. The substitution, however, must be appropriate. An example of an inappropriate substitution might be blowing a whistle in school when someone steals your client's snack.

dialogue of every character, with prompts from the clinician, without censoring. The play is then acted out, as written, with the child choosing whichever role he or she wants to play.

The second part of this exercise is to brainstorm with the child to come up with a "code phrase" that he or she is to use instead of yelling. The play is re-enacted again, with the child using the code phrase that he or she is to use instead of yelling.

Provided below is an actual script written by an 11-year-old client. We agreed that the code phrase would be "the bell." The script was acted, then re-enacted with the child using the "the bell" in a sentence as a response to parental dialogue. The parent observes the play and he or she is counseled to use a hug (or other positive reinforcement) instead of yelling when the new phrase is produced quietly at home, rewarding the child for the new behavior.

The Exercise

1. Elicit a play from the child. In the following sample script, the questions are written sequentially, but in an actual dialogue, discussion occurs after each question.

   "I want you to think about an event or a situation in which there was a lot of yelling going on. Now let's make up a little play about the situation. Tell me where it happened. Who was there? What were they wearing? What was your first line? Then what did mom say?"

   Continue your dialogue with the child until the script is complete. Following is a sample script as actually written by an 11-year-old voice client.

   ### The Sample Script: Morning at the Hewlett House

   ### The Characters:

   <u>Dad</u> (wearing his suit without a jacket, balding, pot belly)

   <u>Mom</u> (blonde, short, in a yellow robe)

   <u>James</u> (11-year-old boy, brown hair, in blue pajama bottoms)

   ### The Scene:

   It's morning time, around 7 AM. Mom has entered James' room and has opened the blinds. James is awake with his eyes closed, enjoying the comfort of his warm, warm bed.

   Mom: "Time to get up James . . . It's time for school."

James (*with his eyes still closed*): "One minute."

Mom leaves the room without bothering James. James is still relaxing. She comes in about 10 minutes later.

Mom: "Get up, James!"

James (*a little louder this time*): "One minute!"

Mom (*starts to leave but then turns and leans over James*): GET UP!

James: ONE MINUTE!

Dad (*from the stairs below*): "James, you better get up or I'm gonna put something on time-out!!"

James: ONE MINUTE!

Dad (*now runs up the stairs and into James' room*): "Not one minute. It's time to go to school (*He scoops James up out of bed*).

James: "Get off of me!!! Get off . . . GET OFF! I was perfectly comfortable and you could of asked nicely and maybe I would have gotten up!"

Dad (*angrily*): "You want something on time-out?"

James (*yelling*): "Fine fine fine FINE!" (*He runs down the stairs mad*).

"DUMMY!!!" (*He shouts at his Dad from the bottom of the stairs*).

2. Act out the play as written.

3. Brainstorm a code phrase to use as replacement for the undesirable vocal behavior, and re-enact the script. The following is a sample script.

> "Now, let's make up a code word or phrase that you can use instead of yelling. How about the phrase "the bell?" We'll do the play again. You practice using the "the bell" in a sentence. You could say "I hear the bell," or "Is that the bell again?" or "Oh, I hear the bell, I better get up." Mom and Dad agree that they will give you a hug every time you use the code phrase in the morning."

4. Act out the play, with the child using the phrase in place of yelling.

Camp Voice

Leah Ross-Kugler

Purposes

- To increase identification and awareness of vocal behaviors.
- To provide a visual cue to decrease vocal volume.

Origin

Summer camp typically involves singing songs, cheering for team-mates, and screaming in "color war," the louder the better, according to tradition. Many children after summer camp are significantly hoarse, with or without lesions on their vocal folds. Before my young clients leave for camp, I create visual cues to help them to be mindful of their voice use while they are away. These clients usually have had a few sessions in which we have worked on finding substitute behaviors for shouting. Most children enjoy drawing and coloring, so the idea of the camp map was created.

Overview

When learning about summer camp plans, I ask the child questions such as: Have you gone to camp before? What the camp is like? What are some of the camp activities? The child is asked to draw at home, in pencil, a map of the camp and bring it in to the next therapy session. If an older sibling has attended and can draw the camp, or a printed map of the camp is available, it can be brought to the session. If the client doesn't know the camp, then I ask the client to draw what it might look like using the activity list. We sometimes do this together. Then the map is color-coded, according to areas at risk for generating phonotrauma. Then, independently, the client identifies areas associated with different vocal loudnesses. The client also chooses which color represents "loud" or "shouting" (many choose *red*, but not all), which color represents "normal talking," and which color would indicate quiet (no talking). The therapist recognizes and guides answers, but doesn't provide the answers.

The Exercise

1. Discuss the map with the child; have crayons ready. (Dialogue guides the child to increase awareness of areas where there

may be chronic use of loud voice, e.g., shouting, yelling, singing.)

> "So this is your camp, how nice! Why don't you show me around? What happens over here? Over here? Great!"

2. Have the child choose the colors that represent a *loud*, *normal*, and *quiet* time.

> "Now let's color this beautiful drawing. Where on this map is it very noisy? Where you do a lot of singing or shouting? (e.g. the mess hall) OK, let's choose a color for *loud*. What color is *'loud'*? Great, color those areas *red*. What other areas are *red*?" (The child chooses and colors.)

3. Continue to identify and color *quiet* areas on the map (e.g., reading room) and areas where there would be average talking (e.g., art room).

> "What color do you think is *quiet*? (Child says, "Blue.") "Great, color the quiet areas blue. And what color is talking but not yelling? Color those areas _____."

4. Have the child post his or her camp map next to his or her bunk or at home on the refridgerator as a reminder of vocal behaviors and at-risk contexts.

Voice Drawing

Leah Ross-Kugler

Purposes

To increase:

- Vocal variety (prosody) in a child's speech.
- The child's understanding of how suprasegmentals can change the meaning of an utterance.

Origin

This is a fun exercise that I've used with children to help them become more aware of prosody, which I often refer to as the "music of the voice." The exercise stems from my background in both music and art.

Overview

In this exercise, a short sentence is "drawn" with a continuous dashed line and dot technique to represent duration, pitch, and loudness. Young children seem to respond intuitively to the drawn sentences, depending on their fine motor and language skills. Sentences and drawings can be increased in complexity according to the client's age and development. For example, a 3-year-old may not be able to draw a long, complex sentence or be able to imagine abstract words, so you would use simple, concrete words. I sometimes use sentences from comics or books that children enjoy, but often I find it easier to use phrases with which they are unfamiliar so that they have no preconceptions. Words and sentences are presented in a hierarchy from simple to complex, single sentences to poems (Shel Silverstein is a good choice). The exercise can also be done with a recording, with both the clinician and client listening and drawing together. All you need is several sheets of paper, lined or unlined, and charcoal (or any single-color medium that can vary easily in one stroke). In the activity, the therapist says a sentence and simultaneously draws the sentence with lines and dots. The words in the sentence can be thin or thick, long or short, dark or light, or high or low on the page. For example, loud words usually are drawn as thicker, darker lines. Words produced with a longer duration ("legato") are drawn as longer lines. Short, fast ("staccato") words can be represented by a dot. High-pitched words are drawn at the top of the page, and low-pitched words on the bottom (see figures for examples).

The Exercise

Begin the exercise with "Let's draw our voices!" and give a brief explanation of the activity. Following are two sample scripts. See the corresponding illlustrations by number.

1. How many different ways can you say "Hi"?

Pretend you're answering the telephone.

Example 1: You are so excited to hear from the caller, you give the caller a big, enthusiastic greeting like, "HAAAAiiiiiii!"

Example 2: Now try a short, brief "Hi."

Example 3: How about a thin, soft sound, almost like you're sad.

Example 4: Say "Hi?" with your voice rising at the end, as if you're not sure who is calling.

Example 5: Say a breathy, flat "Hi" as though you are sick or weak.

The exercise may be expanded in various ways. The client can finger trace "mountains" and dots while producing one of the utterances. The client can guess which sentence goes with a particular picture. The therapist can hold a contest to see how many different ways a sentence can be drawn. The therapist can start with a line drawing (no words), and see if the client can put words to it. For homework, ask the client to record an interview of a parent, and, in the next session, draw the parent's voice (preset answers may be given to the parent).

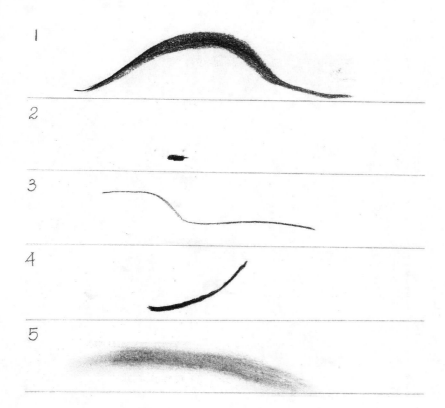

2. How many different ways can you say, "I'll do it"?

Do you mean something different each time you say it?

Example 6: Sound very enthusiastic, like you're eagerly volunteering for something, such as "I'LL do it!"

Example 7: Say it as if you're annoyed.

Example 8: Say it as though you mean, "Quit nagging me!" such as, "I'll DO it!"

Example 9: Now try a breathy, weak voice, as if you don't really want to do it.

Blowing Bubbles

Leah Ross-Kugler

Purposes

- To increase breath control and support
- To facilitate evenflow phonation
- To reduce hyperfunction of the vocal folds.

Origin

This idea developed from several sources and disciplines: voice science, singing lessons, and swimming. I used Ingo Titze's semioccluded vocal tract exercises and combined them with breath work, specifically exhaling/phonating continuously and slowly. I learned great support technique from my old singing teacher, who enabled me to sing long vocal lines on one breath. According to her, swimming was the best exercise for breath support. When swimming, the impedance of the water slowed my exhalation. On certain rhythmic strokes, I would hum while I exhaled in the water.

Overview

I use this exercise with both children and adults, as the goals are the same. Because blowing bubbles is visible, you can "see" the rate and evenness of your exhalation. As a result, clients understand instantly what "evenflow" means. You don't need a swimming pool, but you will need a cup filled about one-third with water and a straw. The exercise begins with simply blowing bubbles (no voicing) and timing it. Then clients are asked to make "smaller" and "steadier" bubbles (no splashing out of the cup!) and time it, trying to increase the duration of bubble-blowing. Then we progress to adding voicing with the straw in the cup. To increase the complexity, this exercise can progress to gently lowering the cup from the straw and gently removing the straw from the lips.

The Exercise

1. Sit upright, bring the straw in the cup to your mouth, maintaining your posture.
2. Inhale deeply and blow into the straw.

3. Time how long you can make bubbles (and keep a record).

4. Inhale deeply and blow into the straw, this time blowing little, tiny bubbles; keep it even (like a "slow boil").

5. Inhale deeply and blow into the straw while voicing (make a sound like uuuuuuuuuuu) into the straw in the water. Try to keep the bubbles tiny and steady.

The Owl

Judith M. Wingate

Purposes

- To teach the concept of high, medium, and low pitches to children.
- To promote use of flow phonation.
- To promote use of easy onset of voice.

Origin

This exercise was inspired by a preschool boy who used a low-pitched and gravelly voice quality to speak. A concrete method for teaching pitch discrimination was needed and this method evolved in the course of therapy.

Overview

This exercise for children teaches pitch discrimination and production using a family of owls. The large owl (papa) has a low-pitched voice, the medium owl (mama) has a mid-pitched voice, and the smallest owl (baby) has a higher pitched voice. The owl makes the sound "whoo" or "hoot." Use of the /u/ vowel allows the child to feel some airflow on a finger held in front of the lips and the initiation of the word with /h/ or /wh/ promotes easy onset of voice. Illustrations of the owls are used to teach the child the difference in the pitch levels and then are used to practice clear voice productions at varying pitch levels. Pitch glides can also be practiced by suggesting that the owls fly up to the tree or down to the ground. Once the child has mastered the use of the appropriate pitch levels, reminders can be given during activities to use one of the pitch targets (such as "Let's try using your baby owl voice right now.").

The Exercise

Introduce the concept of pitch using the owl family pictures. Following is a sample script to use with the child.

The large owl is Papa Owl and he says "whoo." This owl is Mama Owl and she says "whoo." Baby Owl says "whoo." Listen. I will make a sound and you point to the owl that makes the sound.

Now let's practice sounding like each of the owls. We're going to put a finger in front of our lips so we can feel the air on our fingers when we make the "whoo" sound. Let's do five Papa owl sounds. Now try five Mama Owl sounds. And now let's make five baby owl sounds.

Now that you can make the owl sounds, let's practice having the owls make sounds while they fly. Let's have one of the owls fly up to their tree. They will sound like this when they fly. (Produce a whoo on upward glide.)

Now one of the owls sees something good to eat on the ground. When the owl flies down to the ground, it sounds like this. (Produce a whoo on downward glide.)

Let's make the owl fly up and down and practice the sounds. Now, see if you can count to five using a voice like Papa Owl, Mama Owl, and Baby Owl. Now play copycat with me and say some words using each of the owl voices.

Birds Talking!

Rita Hersan

Purpose

- To promote dynamic balance of airflow and voicing.
- To facilitate vocal fold elongation and minimize vocal fold impact stress.
- To motivate children to engage in "voice work."

Origin

Repetition, although considered essential for learning a target vocal behavior, may represent a challenge for children, who often demonstrate lack of interest in and poor motivation for voice therapy. In my experience, having the child play an active role in the voice therapy process as "co-creator" of a vocal technique promotes positive involvement and increases motivation. For example, I often encourage them to come up with meaningful titles for the techniques that are tailored to address their voice problem. "Birds Talking," which exemplifies the notion of co-creativity, spontaneously emerged during a voice therapy session with a seven-year-old child. I have incorporated the exercise into therapy ever since.

Overview

Children who speak with a pressed voice, produced with strong medial compression of the vocal folds, may have increased risk of phonotrauma. Our goal is to engage children to produce voice as safely as possible. Voiced lip and tongue trills have been described as excellent tools to achieve appropriate balance of speech-breathing support, if done on a comfortable pitch and loudness, maintaining minimal effort while producing a buzzy sound. Children usually master lip and tongue trills easily, and, often, they associate the buzz sound to a familiar object such as jackhammer, blender, or motorboat. Children also like to incorporate gestures and body movement while producing lip or tongue buzzes. The exercise normally progresses with pitch glides, which serve as the foundation for conversational speech.

Sample Dialogues

Here are samples of dialogues created by some of my clients.

Initial Dialogue

- Hi! What is your name?
- My name is Zuzu.
- What are you doing Zuzu?
- I am looking for food!
- Follow me, I will show you a special place.
- Wait! What's your name?
- My name is Windy!

Situational Dialogue (See Step 5 in The Exercise)

Feeling frustrated: **Can't play today!**

- What's wrong Windy?
- I can't play today.
- Why not?
- I have to watch my little brothers.
- Where are they?

Feeling scared: **I saw a snake!**

- Zuzu I saw a snake today!
- Really? Where?
- I was eating some seeds on the ground.
- How big was it?
- Too big for me!
- What color?
- Yellow and green.
- Are you scared?
- I am! I will never go back there.

The Exercise

1. Ask the child to help you create a simple dialogue between two birds that have just met.
2. Write the short sentences and make sure that some questions are included, for example: "Hi! What is your name?"
3. Without saying the words, and producing **only** lip or tongue trills, simulate the dialogue using all the appropriate pitch inflection that was present in the original script.
4. Make sure the child pauses and uses pitch variation that is easy and not strained. If necessary, use negative practice producing pressed versus easy lip or tongue trills.
5. Create different situations for different dialogues during each session. When practicing *Birds Talking*, children will also be able to express different feelings such as sadness, happiness, boredom, excitement, tiredness, anger, or fear, depending on how they produce downward and upward inflections associated with gesture and facial expression.
6. For transferring *Birds Talking* to real speech, use the original dialogue and ask the child to feel easy voicing while emphasizing the inflections.

Note: Allow the child to repeat your pitch inflection if he or she feels shy about initiating the exercise. Loudness variation can also be included.

Chapter 11

SPECIAL CASES

Throughout this book, our approach has not been to direct exercises to specific disorders. Some voice disorders, however, need to be approached differently. Here we present a few of those special cases in voice therapy.

Six special groups of clients are addressed in this chapter: transgender clients, those who are diagnosed with mutational falsetto, paradoxical vocal fold motion, functional aphonia, vocal tremor, and clients whose occupation requires speaking to groups or giving prepared presentations.

Four exercises are offered for those working with transgender clients. Heuer's *Modification of Pitch in Male-to-Female Transgendered Clients* uses visual feedback to help clients become accustomed to using a higher pitch range. His exercise also addresses the linguistic content of a client's utterances, so that the client can practice a more feminized style of speaking in addition to using a higher pitch. Pickering and Kayajian's *Modifying Frequency and Resonance in Individuals Who Are Transgender* combines a resonant voice therapy approach with an adaptation of Stemple's Vocal Function Exercises to achieve a functional pitch change in this group of clients. Block is represented by two exercises: *Chant Your Pitch* (for a transfeminine voice) which uses a resonance approach, focusing on chanting and training the target pitch, and *Count Big* (for voice masculinization), which has the goal of a "bigger voice" for clients who want to achieve a more masculine voice.

Pitch is also the focus of therapy for clients with puberphonia, the persistence of an immature pitch in young adult men. Yiu's *Cough or Throat-Clear Phonation for Puberphonia* targets mutational falsetto in young men. A gentle cough or throat-clear is used to initiate brief phonation by taking advantage of the low tension, and hence low pitch, produced by these vegetative maneuvers. The resulting sound is then extended and shaped into other sounds and phrases at the target pitch.

This chapter also addresses therapy for individuals with abnormal muscular activity: paradoxical vocal fold motion and functional aphonia. The four exercises for paradoxical vocal fold motion

(PVFM), also called vocal cord dysfunction, seek to remove the excessive muscular activity of the chest and larynx that many consider to underlie this disorder. Blager, in *Relaxed Throat Breathing*, uses a voiceless fricative with focus on abdominal muscle control to help the client achieve normal breathing. The new breathing pattern is then incorporated into walking and other physical activity. Murry, in *Low Resistance Rhythmic Breathing for Paradoxical Vocal Fold Motion*, uses walking at the start of the exercise to help establish a normal rhythmic breathing pattern for the client, thereby diminishing excessive inhalations. Gherson's *Paradoxical Vocal Fold Motion Rescue Strategies* uses four techniques: quick sniff, tongue pull-backs, a tripartite "stop, drop, and roll" drill, and breathing pacing, all towards slowing down and then reversing the procession of PVFM symptoms. Litt and Gartner-Schmidt's *Training Open Orolaryngopharyngeal Postures* for PVFMD uses the image of the vocal tract as an open tube to help the client minimize orolaryngeal tension that accompanies PFVM.

Many therapists successfully address functional aphonia using Roy's techniques that require physical manipulation of the client's larynx. In this chapter, Spencer's *Hands-Off Treatment for Functional Aphonia* offers an approach for clients who cannot tolerate physical manipulation. This exercise provides an excellent example of how diverse approaches can better meet the needs of our diverse client population.

This chapter also includes an exercise for clients with vocal tremor. Although voice therapy cannot remove the tremor, Barmkeier-Kraemer's *Hiding Vocal Tremor* capitalizes upon compensatory strategies, including staccato-style speaking, to minimize the perceptual manifestation of the tremor.

Finally, Behrman's *Conversational Voice Therapy* is designed for clients such as teachers, public speakers, sales people, trainers, and others who give frequent formal presentations. The series of exercises, serving a preventive purpose, draws upon public speaking techniques to minimize voice disorders that can arise if speakers misuse their voice when addressing audiences.

As always, we remind the reader that the exercises provided in this chapter are not the only ones that may be successful with the client populations that are targeted here. Peruse other chapters for exercises, some of which you may find are appropriate to use "as is," and others that you may want to adapt to your client's specific needs.

Modification of Pitch in Male-to-Female Transgendered Clients

Reinhardt Heuer

Purpose

■ To raise the average speaking pitch level in male-to-female transgendered clients.

Origin

In my experience, two issues are central to working with male-to-female transgendered clients. First, pitch is the communicative feature of which they are most aware and which they are most sensitive to changing, regardless of whether the pitch level is actually a problem. Second, many of my clients do not discriminate well between different pitches when producing the sounds themselves. Therefore, I have found that use of visual cues can be quite helpful, followed by auditory training to fade the cues as we work to transfer the new pitch to spontaneous speech.

Overview

For visual feedback, I use the Real Pitch Program (Kay Elemetrics Corp., Lincoln Park, NJ). The older version of the program, the Visi-Pitch, as well as many software products from other sources can also be used. One software system, PRAAT, can be downloaded from the Internet at no charge, and can be used by your clients for home practice.

I set the baseline pitch on the computer at 155 Hz, which appears to be approximately the frequency below which people perceive the voice to be male, and above which people perceive the voice to be female. The client produces utterances in response to the clinician's questions, and the goal is for the client to keep the pitch of the entire utterance well above 155 Hz. Another option is to set the baseline lower than 155 Hz, and then gradually raise it as the client achieves success with the new pitch.

Note: For training and home practice material, I recommend using phrases that the client develops herself, in part because the material would then be most relevant to the client. In addition, it provides an opportunity to work on modifying the content toward a more culturally feminine wording.

The Exercise

It is important that the client achieve the higher pitch without strain. The therapist may find it necessary to incorporate relaxation, breathing, and resonance exercises at the higher pitch to help the client achieve the new voice efficiently and easily.

1. Start by keeping a diary of phrases that you use during the week. The diary will enable you to practice changing your pitch and feminizing your language using sentences that come from your actual conversations. (Recording telephone calls is a good way to observe words and phrases that you typically use, although you will probably want to tell your conversational partner that the call is being recorded.)

2. Discuss your diary in the therapy sessions, toward the goal of identifying utterances that appear to have masculine wording. Develop alternative wordings that sound more feminine.

3. In the sessions, using the software program, practice saying the revised phrases from your diary, trying to keep your pitch far enough above the baseline so that you can use a pitch pattern of four tones, all of which are above the baseline. Audio-record your practice, so that you can use the recording as a guide for the target pitch when you practice at home. (Alternatively, if available to you, you can use a software program of your own.) If you are experiencing difficulty raising your pitch comfortably to the target level, first practice gliding your pitch upward in a relaxed manner.

4. After you have achieved success in using your new pitch and feminine phrasing with your practice sentences, practice with other material, including reading and conversation.

5. As you become more comfortable using your new pitch with a variety of spoken material, your goal is to decrease your dependence on visual feedback. Practice without looking at the computer screen. After you say one or more phrases, make a judgment about the appropriateness of your pitch, and then look at the computer screen to check your accuracy. As your accuracy increases, your confidence will increase and your speech will become more spontaneous at the new pitch.

Modifying Frequency and Resonance for Individuals Who Are Transgender

Jack Pickering and Daniel Kayajian

Purposes

- To safely increase or decrease the fundamental frequency for an individual who is transgender
- To produce fundamental frequency and resonance that are consistent with an individual's gender identity
- To improve vocal balance and flexibility, facilitate forward resonatory focus, and reduce vocal effort
- To help individuals who are transgender gain confidence as they modify their communication skills.

Origin

Recently, speech-language pathologists have become increasingly involved in voice and communication modification for people who are transgender. Changing fundamental frequency and resonance are key ways of facilitating appropriate gender perception for transgender individuals. Although other aspects of communication are important (e.g., nonverbal communication, language, projection), changing frequency and resonance are important foundational activities in therapy. In our group program, we use Vocal Function Exercises (VFEs), as described by Stemple (2010), and aspects of Resonant Voice Therapy (RVT), as described by Verdolini-Marston, Burke, Lessac, Glaze, and Caldwell (1995), to facilitate vocal balance and flexibility, forward resonatory focus, and reduced vocal effort. These approaches were selected because they have been shown to be effective with clients who have voice disorders, and allow us to change fundamental frequency and resonance in a systematic, safe way, while also facilitating client confidence. For clients who are transitioning from male to female (MtF), we attempt to increase frequency; for clients transitioning from female to male (FtM), we attempt to decrease frequency. The way we use these approaches will be the same for both client groups. The following overview and exercise description is for individuals transitioning from male to female, since we work with considerably more MtF clients. And although we use these exercises in our group transgender program, they are described below for an individual therapy session.

Overview

Prior to performing the two exercises, our transgender clients take part in mindfulness or relaxation in the very beginning of each session, followed by some easy vocalizations to warm up (humming, straw phonation, "molms"). Clients warm up on a note that is consistent with a female voice (e.g., F3, G3, A3), so they can begin experiencing a vocal pitch that will match their gender identity. We are flexible in selecting the type of vocalization, and often experiment to find the vocalization that works best for each individual.

After warming up, clients complete VFEs using one of three ranges: C3–G3 (baritone), E3–B3 (tenor), or A3–E4 (alto). The range for each client is chosen after probing for the client's average fundamental frequency during a prolonged vowel and counting. Estill Voice International's Voiceprint is used to determine average fundamental frequency; we have also used a KayPentax VisiPitch. Once the average fundamental frequency is determined, clients try the VFE range that is just higher than the range typically applied for clients with voice disorders. It is anticipated that clients will perform VFEs at one range for 6 to 8 weeks. Most MtF clients can accomplish VFEs at E3–A3, even if they were males perceived to have a very low pitch; some clients can reach the alto range of A3–E4.

After 3 to 4 weeks working on VFEs, aspects of Resonant Voice Therapy (RVT) are incorporated into the program in order to focus attention on resonance (see Stemple's VFEs in this volume). We find that RVT provides a good context for focusing on inflection and facilitating forward tone focus in connected speech (see the exercises on increasing resonance in this volume). Eliminating back focused resonance and the accompanying glottal fry is particularly useful for MtF clients.

Consistent with RVTs, our first activity attempts to establish vibration in the front of the mouth, the lips, teeth, gums, and so forth. Once our clients establish forward vibration and tone, we tend to use the mo-mo-mo posture (or molm, as described by Stemple) to practice producing forward tone focus in subsequent steps. As we follow the steps, feedback is provided on resonance, as well as breathing, voice quality, and the "female-ness" of the voice. Speaking in molm is fun and a good jumping-off point for our clients to produce connected speech.

The Exercises

Adapted VFEs

There are 4 steps to the VFEs. Do them twice each day, once in the morning and once in the evening. Use a piano, pitch pipe, or iPad app to produce and match each note.

1. To warm up, sustain a twangy /i/ for as long as possible on the musical note F3 (for the baritone range), or A3 (for the tenor range), or D4 (for the alto range). Do this twice and record your time on each production.
2. Stretching. Glide from your most comfortable low note to the highest note on the word "knoll" or "whoop" or during a lip trill. Do this twice. Produce the glides with buzzing lips; your goal is to glide without a voice break.
3. Contracting. For this next exercise, glide from your most comfortable high note to the lowest note on the word "knoll" or "whoop" or during a lip trill. Do this twice. Produce the glides with buzzing lips; your goal is to glide without a voice break. When you get down low, don't let your voice fall back in your throat and sound gravelly.
4. To increase your power, sustain each of the five musical notes in your range (e.g., E3-F3-G3-A3-B3 for the tenor range) for as long as possible with good lip buzz on the word "old" without the /d/. Produced each of these notes twice and record your times.

Adapted RVT

For RVT, focus on producing vibration in your lips, face, inside your mouth, something called forward tone focus. Like the VFEs, use a pitch pipe, piano, or iPad app to produce and match notes that are consistent with a female voice (F3, G3, A3). Practice this exercise for a short time each day, especially before speaking in public.

1. You start RVT by humming, saying hum-um-um, phonating with a straw, or molming using a chant, which ever helps you produce the best vibration in your lips, face, inside your mouth. Also, notice the limited effort in your throat during these productions.
2. Now produce syllable strings (molm-molm-molm, me-me-me, moo-moo-moo, or ma-ma-ma) as a sigh. Then try them with varying rate (slow-fast-slow) and loudness (soft-loud-soft) on your most comfortable female note, F3, G3, or A3.
3. Produce molm-molm-molm (or other syllable string) in a speech-like way, varying inflection as if you are asking questions and making statements. Try to maintain your best female voice.
4. Next, produce voiced sentences loaded with /m/ or /n/ sounds (Mari made me mad; My momma made marmalade; Nelly needs Nana now), first as a chant, then with overexaggerated inflection (lots of excitement), and finally as natural speech.
5. In the next step, produce voiced/voiceless sentences (My mom put Pete on the moon; Pete and Paul made mom mad), first as a chant, then with exaggerated inflection, and finally like natural speech.

> Clients are carefully monitored during the first two sessions to make sure they are not straining, and if so, their range is adjusted down, even by a note or two. Over time, clients also attempt higher notes, in case they might be able to move up to a new range.

> Glides up and down the scale can help with gender appropriate pitch change. Glides down the scale can also help individuals understand forward versus back tone focus, by explaining that pitch can be decreased without letting the voice fall back in the throat.

> A picture of a piano keyboard is used to show clients their starting average frequency and where they need to go in order to be perceived as female. This has been particularly helpful for clients who are not musically inclined.

> We often start RVTs by using the analogy of the flute and piccolo, suggesting that we are trying to make the flute (a longer, male vocal tract) sound like a piccolo (a shorter, female vocal tract) using these activities.

> Many MtF transgender individuals struggle to project their voice once they attain a female or gender-neutral fundamental frequency. Producing soft-loud-soft molms on F3, G3, or A3 provides a way to help transgender clients project their voice in a safe, effective, and gender-appropriate way.

6. After producing these sentences, try more complicated sentences and do some paragraph reading. Finally, try using your new skills in conversation. Focus on using your best female voice.

Chant Your Pitch (Voice Feminization)

Christie Block

Purposes

- To increase average pitch
- To maintain a higher average pitch
- To increase forward resonance
- To prevent laryngeal tension.

Origin

Higher pitch is commonly understood to be a critical component of a feminine voice, and pitch is where I typically begin my work with transsexual, transgender, and gender nonconforming clients who seek to attain a more feminine presentation. I learned to use chant-to-talk exercises for voice rehabilitation as a graduate student, and I have come to utilize them when introducing a target pitch in a healthy way. My version of chant-to-talk for voice feminization focuses on chanting a target pitch and then aiming higher than that pitch at the onset of speech. This allows for a clear target pitch as well as freedom of pitch movement within a natural range. By initially aiming higher than the chant, the client is more likely to achieve the targeted average, yet not overshoot by staying within an intuitive intonation range around the target. My focus on aiming high at onset across utterances was inspired by a demonstration by Mary Tish Moody SLP with a transfeminine client at a Voice Foundation Symposium.

Overview

This exercise elicits a target average pitch of G3 (196 Hz), which is one tone higher than "gender ambiguous" pitch (see Adler et al., 2006 for discussion and literature review). The target pitch may be 1 to 2 tones higher or lower than G3, and, if lower, may increase one to two tones from the initial target, depending on individual needs. The exercise starts with a hum in order to tune to the target pitch and achieve relaxed forward resonance. Then, the client is trained to chant then count, advancing to more difficult linguistic levels. The client may need to hum periodically at the target pitch as the exercise progresses. Pitch range and specific feminine-identified intonation contours are also introduced if necessary.

> Pitch feedback tools are often useful initially during sessions and home practice. A guitar tuner or piano keyboard—in the form of hardware, Web sites, or phone apps—can model and check the pitch of a sustained tone (hum). Software programs such as Real-Time Pitch from KayPentax or VoicePrint from Estill Voice International Inc. provide visual feedback during connected speech with an adjustable reference pitch.

Note: The client is encouraged to hum the target pitch during routine activities such as waking up, going to bed, taking a shower, and so forth.

The Exercise

1. Say /m/ at G3 for 2 to 3 seconds 10 times.
2. Say /m/ at G3 once for 2 to 3 seconds. Then count in a chant at G3: 1-2-3-4 breath 5-6-7-8 breath 9-10-11-12 breath 13-14-15-16 breath 17-18-19-20.
3. Say /m/ at G3 once for 2 to 3 seconds. Then count in a speaking voice, starting higher than G3 at the beginning of each set of four numbers: 1-2-3-4 breath 5-6-7-8 breath 9-10-11-12 breath 13-14-15-16 breath 17-18-19-20.
4. Chant a sentence at G3, then say the sentence starting higher than G3.
5. Chant a sentence at G3, then say the sentence starting higher than G3. Then make up another sentence to go with it starting higher than G3.
6. Read a passage. Start higher than G3 at the beginning of every sentence or phrase.

Count Big (Voice Masculinization)

Christie Block

Purposes

- To increase loudness
- To increase linking of sounds and words
- To increase articulatory movement
- To increase open oral resonance
- To prevent laryngeal tension.

Origin

A lower pitch, even when aided by testosterone, can be insufficient for transsexual, transgender, and gender nonconforming people who aim to express themselves in a more masculine way. One of the non-pitch components of my voice masculinization work focuses on the concept of a "bigger voice," which maximizes the size of the oral-pharyngeal space and draws upon the power of the vocal mechanism that the client biologically possesses. I have adapted rehabilitative voice techniques that typically address hyperfunction and hypernasality to help the transmasculine client increase awareness and accuracy of a richer sound in a natural and healthy way.

Overview

This exercise elicits an increasingly "bigger voice" through increased linking, loudness, articulatory movement, and open oral resonance. In this way, the client becomes aware of a number of ways to achieve a richer sound, progressing from commonly familiar concepts to less familiar ones. /m/-initial syllables are integrated into the exercise so that laryngeal tension is prevented as the size of the oral and pharyngeal cavities increase. This exercise can serve as a quick periodic boost as well as an introduction to more intensive oral resonance practice, such as the use of minimal pairs comparing low versus high vowels and/or back versus front vowels, with advancement to higher linguistic levels.

In this exercise, "full voice" means linked, connected, or blended phonation, and slightly increased loudness level. "Big/bigger voice" means full voice, as above, as well as open mouth, and open throat, resulting in increased linking, loudness level, articulatory movement, and open oral resonance.

The Exercise

1. Count from 1 to 5 two times in a full voice by linking the numbers and increasing the loudness level slightly. Take a relaxed breath between each set.
2. Again, count from 1 to 5 two times, this time with a bigger sound, combining a full voice with a more open mouth. Notice your lips moving freely, and allow your jaw to lower slightly on every number. You should be able to achieve this sound without increasing your loudness further.
3. Yawn with a sigh ("ha!") three times. Notice your throat opening up now in addition to your mouth.
4. Say /ma-ma-ma-mi-mi-mi/ three times, exaggerating the bigger sound of /ma/ (open mouth and throat) compared to the smaller sound of /mi/ (nearly closed mouth and throat).
5. Repeat Step 4, making /mi/ sound bigger like /ma/, keeping your mouth and throat open with a low, relaxed jaw and base-of-tongue.
6. Again, count from 1 to 5 two times with an even bigger sound than when counting before, combining all three components of full voice, open mouth, and open throat.
7. Count from 1 to 5 six times by repeating steps 1, 2, and 6 consecutively, achieving an increasingly bigger sound with each step.

Relaxed Throat Breathing

Florence B. Blager

Purpose

■ To facilitate normal breathing in clients with vocal fold dysfunction.

Origin

I developed the Relaxed Throat Breathing technique in 1982, when vocal fold dysfunction was first recognized at National Jewish Medical and Research Center. When asked if I could do something to help these patients, I realized that they were showing a maladaptive pattern similar to patients with functional voice disorders. Results of our success using this approach were published in *The New England Journal of Medicine* (Christopher, Wood, Eckert, Blager, Raney, & Souhrada, 1983).

Overview

We believe that clients with vocal fold dysfunction, when experiencing upper airway constriction, attempt to breathe by focusing on where the constriction is perceived. As a result, the upper chest, shoulders, external laryngeal structures, and intrinsic laryngeal muscles all become overengaged in the attempt to release the upper airway constriction, and allow air once again to move freely through the airway. In contrast, the conceptual model of Relaxed Throat Breathing focuses on the breath and allows the air to move freely as though from the abdomen or rib cage up to and through "the mask" (the front of the oral/nasal cavities) without using the larynx to help move the air. To achieve this relaxation, the therapist can have the client focus on abdominal support. Alternatively, if the client has difficulty achieving appropriate abdominal movement, the focus can be shifted to the rib cage, and then to feeling the air movement through the lips. After learning to focus on the lips and mouth, clients frequently will let go of effortful upper muscle support for the breath, and move into use of the abdomen.

Note: Throughout the practice, the therapist should help the client to internalize the concept that stridor or the sensation of tightness while breathing can be released by performing this exercise.

The Exercises

Part I. Basic Relaxed Throat Breathing

1. Take a "relaxed throat breath." Keep your tongue on the floor of your mouth with your lips gently closed, and gently release your jaw.
2. Place a finger on your lips and exhale on a gentle /s/ with abdominal support. Alternatively, you may use /ʃ/ or /f/ if these sounds give you a stronger sensation of the breath moving through your mouth and lips.
3. Then, to feel the breath support, put your hand on your abdomen. You should feel the abdomen expand as you inhale, and move inward as you exhale.
4. Perform five of these breaths regularly on the following schedule:

   - In the morning
   - At noon
   - Before bedtime
   - Before medications
   - As it fits into your schedule

   In addition, at the first sign of tightness or stridor, stop what you are doing and perform this breathing exercise. Always perform the exercise easily: don't push or pull on your shoulders, chest, or neck. Concentrate on letting air in and out. When the stridor stops, gradually resume the activity.

5. Go into new activities and sports gradually, using the breath as a basic part of your activity.

Part II. Activity-Based Breathing

With younger clients as well as with adults involved in active sports, the breathing pattern should be adapted by moving the focus from the abdomen up to the rib cage. This focus allows for a more rapid inhale and exhale. Each sport has a specific body pattern which needs to be analyzed with the client. For example, basketball requires quick, rapid changes of direction at rapid speed whereas soccer requires extended running at a rapid speed, with stops and starts. The new breathing pattern needs to be integrated into the body pattern by slowing down the pace of the sport.

Note: If the client is an athlete, you will need space (school gym or playing field) to expand the breathing techniques into a movement pattern for a particular sport. The following is just a sample of the stages of application of the "relaxed throat breath" described in Part I. As noted above, the focus is now on the rib cage expanding with the inhalation and contracting with the exhalation.

1. Stand in place. Focus on the breathing technique.
2. Walk in place. Maintain the breathing coordination.
3. Walk across the floor slowly with your hands on your rib cage. Increase the pace of your walking. Remove your hands from your rib cage. If you are unable to maintain breathing from the rib cage without using your hands, reduce your pace and return to using your hands.
4. Jog slowly across the floor. Inhale and exhale using gently pursed lips. Place your hands on your rib cage if necessary. Alternate walking with jogging until a slow jog across the floor can be maintained without having your hands on your rib cage.
5. Increase the pace of the jogging. Expect the pace of the inhale and the exhale to increase as the pace of the jog increases. If loss of breathing pattern and/or a sensation of constriction occurs, slow your pace until the correct breathing pattern can be re-established.
6. Increase your exertion level. Start with the pace of a jog at which Activity-Based Breathing can be maintained. Continue the pattern of increasing the pace for brief periods, reducing the pace, and increasing the pace while the breathing pattern is maintained. Your goal is to aim for high exertion levels for longer periods, while maintaining the correct breathing pattern.
7. When you are able to maintain the correct breathing pattern consistently, practice in other settings, for example, while walking or jogging at a school track or at a nearby park.

> *Cautionary Note:* When you work with adolescent athletes, remember (a) adolescents are going through a growth period; (b) the body that used to work spontaneously is not responding in the old patterns; and (c) it may require a long period for the adolescent athlete to integrate the new body with the skills of the sport. Avoid making promises to any client about the level of performance that could be achieved as a result of therapy.

Low-Resistance Rhythmic Breathing for Paradoxical Vocal Fold Motion

Thomas Murry

Purposes

- To inhibit excessive laryngeal tension and abnormal vocal fold movement prior to onset of phonation.
- To relax the upper chest muscles.

Origin

This exercise is a variation of one of several exercises described by Florence Blager some years ago when discussing treatment for paradoxical vocal fold motion. (See the exercise by Florence Blager in this chapter.) One of Dr. Blager's approaches is to reduce tension in the upper chest muscles so that the shoulders do not elevate or rotate forward prior to phonation. By maintaining a relaxed upper chest, it is hypothesized that the client can use less air pressure for phonation. I have observed that clients with documented paradoxical vocal fold motion often complain that they begin to cough or feel short of breath after talking for only a minute or two. When I have observed their conversational speech, I have noted short, shallow inhalations, shoulder elevation on inhalation, and sighing after a short sentence or two. I have used the technique described below with considerable success with clients with paradoxical vocal fold motion.

Overview

This exercise uses rhythmic breathing to decrease the tension in the upper chest muscles and shoulders, in particular, prior to speaking, and to achieve normal breathing. The exercise begins with low resistance breathing in the absence of phonation. The client is guided to inhale through the nose and exhale through the mouth throughout the exercise.

Note: This exercise is to be used only with clients diagnosed with paradoxical vocal fold motion. It will seem unnatural and unnecessary to anyone without this disorder.

The Exercise

1. Walk down a short hallway or across a large room as you breathe out through your mouth. You do not have to force the breath out. Use a natural breath with your mouth open. After you breathe out, close your mouth. Stay in rhythm as you breathe. You do not have to take a breath in to start; you have more than a liter of air in your lungs without inhaling.

2. Walk slowly down the hallway (or across the room) and on every fourth step exhale smoothly and evenly. Do not blow the air out and do not force it through a narrow slit in the lips. This plan is diagrammed below.

R	L	R	L	R
Exhale				Exhale
Mouth open	-------------------	Mouth closed	---------------	Mouth open
1	2	3	4	1

> If the client is having some difficulty staying in rhythm, the therapist can count: 1, 2, 3, 4. The therapist can also ask the client to swing his or her arms gently while walking. Clients with extreme tension hold their arms rigid while walking. Learning to achieve a smooth and rhythmic breathing pattern while walking may occupy an entire therapy session.

Relax your shoulders before starting to walk. Start with an exhalation. Do not take a breath in—even a short, catch breath before the first step. Begin walking more slowly than you usually walk. Walk for approximately 30 to 40 seconds. If you are not forcing the air out on exhalation, then you should not feel the need for big inhalations. Perhaps you felt the air coming back in through your nose, although that is not necessary. Do not progress to the next step until you are able to do the exercise in rhythm and without breath holding.

3. After you achieve a smooth and stable rhythm while walking, sit down in a chair, but do not lean back. Perform the breathing exercise again while sitting. Start without inhaling. You can tap out the rhythmic count with your hands or feet. Always stay in rhythm and always start the exercise on exhalation. (diagram below) Now that you are sitting down, you should feel the air slowly coming in through your nose on the second, third and fourth counts. After you have achieved success in the rhythm and location of the breath, shift to breathing in and out through the nose using the same rhythm pattern.

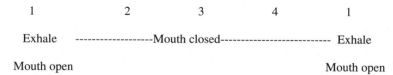

1	2	3	4	1
Exhale	------------------	Mouth closed	-------------------------	Exhale
Mouth open				Mouth open

4. Now try saying a word while exhaling as you walk. It can be helpful to select words that begin with /w/ so that you can feel the air as you start the word. Continue to make sure that you do not take in short "catch" breaths prior to the exhalation. (Refer to diagram below) Ask yourself if you can feel when the air, or breath, is coming into your throat. Place one hand below the base of your sternum and feel movement of the abdominal muscles on inhalation.

R	L	R	L	R
Exhale				Exhale
Mouth open	--------------------Mouth closed----------------			Mouth open
ONE				ONE

5. Continue to practice talking on exhalation, progressing to short phrases and then sentences. Always start phonation without an inhalation.

6. Optional: Modify the rhythm to a pattern that allows you to exhale on every step of your right foot and inhale on every step of your left foot. As always, start slowly and then gradually increase your speed.

Paradoxical Vocal Fold Motion (PVFM) Rescue Strategies

Shirley Gherson

Purposes

- To reverse or slow down the progression of PVFM symptoms.
- To facilitate a return to coordinated, relaxed breathing.
- To reduce excessive tension associated with a PVFM episode.

Origin

I started using this series of exercises while working with athletes and other high level performers, who needed to regain control of their breathing during a game quickly. The concepts behind these strategies are taken mainly from the work of Florence Blager (see her exercise in this volume) and are heavily influenced by Mary J. Sandage, PhD, who discusses the concept of breath recovery in many of her publications on the subject.

Overview

A PVFM episode causes, in many cases, an overwhelming sense of restricted breathing or tightness at the level of the larynx. These rescue strategies may be implemented both as diversion tactics, to shift the focus of control away from the larynx, and as a therapeutic maneuvers to train more appropriate respiratory coordination. The laryngeal lowering techniques (sniffs and tongue pull-back) engage the sensation of a wide-open throat. The associated oropharyngeal posture reduces resistance to inhalation. Elongated exhalations noted in the "Stop, Drop, and Roll" and "Breath-Pacing" exercises below encourage a more natural, passive inhalation.

Clients should be instructed to practice these exercises five times per day or more. This intense practice regimen allows for motor programming and a high comfort and confidence level, when using the technique at the spur of the moment. During a PVFM attack, a client may use one or a combination of rescue strategies, and will likely need to slow down to focus on breath coordination.

Note: In the moment of a PVFM attack, a client's instinct is to struggle against an already tense larynx, often intensifying the symptoms. In training, therapists should be acutely aware of tendencies to overbreathe with the stress of persistent respiratory tension. It may be helpful for the client to start at the end of a comfortable exhalation.

The Exercises

Quick Sniffs

1. Following a comfortable exhale, engage a short and quick sniff three times in rapid succession. Notice the sensation of a tug in the throat or a brief lowering of the larynx. This should feel like a wide-open throat sensation. Pay attention to the sound of the sniff through your nostrils. Repeat this series five times.
2. Transition into two short sniffs followed by one long drawn-out sniff. Be sure to monitor the sensation of laryngeal lowering and listen to the turbulent sound of sniffing through your nose.

Tongue Pull-Back

1. Pull-back the tongue in an "R" posture and feel the lowering of the larynx.
2. Hold the tongue in this position while slowly breathing in and out two or three times.
3. Release the tongue and swallow.
4. Repeat steps 1 through 3 up to five times.

Stop, Drop, and Roll

> **Recap**
>
> ■ **Stop** what you are doing
> ■ **Drop** your tension
> ■ **Roll** out your breath on a lip trill or sustained "ssss."

1. The first part of Stop, Drop, and Roll is to stop or slow down the activity that is triggering an attack. This allows you to focus your attention to your breath.
2. Now focus on the tense areas of the body, such as the jaw, shoulders, or abdomen, and work to release the tension. This is the "drop" part of the exercise.
3. Finally, use a lip trill or sustained "sss" to roll out the breath to reset the body for a relaxed and passive inhale.

Breath Pacing

1. Use the strides of your walk or slow jog to count out a prolonged exhalation followed by an inhalation. Repeat this several times until the pace feels comfortable and the numbers feel steady.
2. Record these numbers when you are not experiencing symptoms and use them as a guide to reinforce a slower, more controlled breath cycle.

Training Open Orolaryngopharyngeal Postures for PVFM

Juliana Litts and Jackie Gartner-Schmidt

Purposes

- To use open orolaryngopharyngeal postures to prevent and rescue clients from upper airway dyspnea related to Paradoxical Vocal Fold Motion Disorder (PVFM)
- To instruct open orolaryngopharyngeal postures that facilitate relief from orolaryngopharyngeal tension and return to unconstricted orolaryngopharyngeal patterns of breathing.

Origin

The following exercises were developed as a variation of Blager's Relaxed Throat Breathing exercises (see her exercise in this volume) that facilitate the reduction of laryngeal tension. Building on knowledge from MRI data that certain oral and laryngeal postures maximize openness in the laryngeal vestibule and posterior pharynx (Story, Titze, & Hoffman, 1996), these exercises integrate tension-relieving upper airway breathing postures for clients with PVFMD.

Overview

The purpose of these exercises is to explicitly change the orolaryngopharyngeal "landscape" to counteract the known effects of a raised larynx and increased medial constriction at the level of the vocal folds during PVFM-related breathing episodes. These lowered-jaw and pursed-lip breathing postures create a series of reactions that allow the extrinsic muscles of the larynx to lower the hyoid bone and in turn lower the larynx. The downward traction of a lowered jaw immediately lengthens the orolaryngopharyngeal tube. The pursed lip and /u/ posture of the oral and pharyngeal cavities has been shown, through MRI data, to create the most wide open posture for the laryngeal vestibule area, decreasing medial constriction at the glottal and supraglottal levels. This action minimizes the anxiety about breathing, which can create muscular constriction in the throat.

Clients are coached using anatomical and physiological references that start during the endoscopic evaluation. In order to facilitate biofeedback, as well as establish a sense of control over their upper airway, clients are asked to visualize the different laryngeal postures between noisy/stridorous inhalation and an open orolaryngopharyngeal posture. Often, clients feel like "victims" of their constricted throat-breathing episodes. Visualizing open versus closed laryngopharyngeal postures during inhalation and exhalation quickly establishes client control. Negative practice is initiated in the first session to improve proprioceptive awareness of open versus closed orolaryngopharyngeal postures. It should be noted that these exercises are not focused on breathing, but rather increased awareness of the proprioceptive sensations of "open versus closed" throat postures while breathing.

Exercises

Prevention of Constricted Upper Airway Postures During Inhalation and Exhalation

Some clients have known triggers to their PVFM-related breathing episodes. In situations where clients may knowingly be exposed to a trigger, *preventing* an attack is key. The following instructions should be used:

> If the client's dyspnea is triggered by exertion, the therapist should instruct the client, using his or her chosen form of exertion or exercise. It is important to note that clients may be required to sign a liability release when therapy is "off site" at certain medical institutions.

1. Think of the mouth and throat as a tube. Relax your shoulders and drop your jaw. This lengthens the tube. Pretend that you are holding a golf ball inside your mouth to facilitate oral openness.
2. Without modifying this posture, inhale and exhale through pursed lips. The inhale should be relatively quick and you should feel the airflow at the lips (e.g., a sip of air). In addition, pretend that you are sucking a thick milkshake through a straw. Exhale slowly with a steady stream of air flowing out pursed lips.
3. Keep an open mouth, and make sure that your exhalation is longer than your inhalation. This should feel like your normal resting breathing pattern. If exhalation is not longer than inhalation, hyperventilation, tingling, or lightheadedness may occur.
4. Continue to pay attention to inhalation and exhalation at the lips until the trigger is reduced.

Rescue Breathing

The prevention breathing exercises mentioned above are not always effective in avoiding the onset of PVFMD-associated episodes. The following instructions should be employed immediately to "rescue" a client from an acute PVFMD attack.

1. Think of your mouth and throat as a tube. Relax your shoulders and drop your jaw to immediately lengthen the tube.

2. Exhale quickly with pursed lips as if you are gently blowing out candles on a cake. Focus on the sensation of steady airflow coming out of the lips.

3. Continue breathing with the pursed lips until the throat constriction has subsided and you have regained control of your upper airway dyspnea.

Practice

1. You should intentionally mimic a "tight throat" breathing posture in contrast with an "open throat" posture. Feel the difference in the location of the feelings of constriction.

2. Once the appropriate upper airway breathing posture has been established, spend time practicing the posture when you are both asymptomatic and symptomatic. The goal is for this posture to become second nature in feeling, so that it is easily accessible when needed.

Hands-Off Treatment for Functional Aphonia

Martin L. Spencer

Purpose

■ To promote resolution of functional aphonia without hands-on laryngeal manipulation.

Origin

This approach was developed to minimize client discomfort, perceived injury, or adverse consequence (e.g., syncope) accompanying circumlaryngeal massage or manual techniques. Over the past decades, laryngeal reposturing and circumlaryngeal massage have become increasingly popular as viable modes of intervention for functional aphonia (FA) and related Muscle Tension Dysphonia (MTD) intervention. The evidence-based success of these methods is largely attributable to the efforts of Arnold Aronson, Nelson Roy, and Jacob Lieberman (see discussion in Roy, Bless, Heisey, & Ford, 1996). I have used these hands-on approaches with success. However, across time I have become wary of sustained manual effort, as the client may perceive it to be harmful, due to the discomfort when performing the maneuvers. A significant benefit of this method is that a client can practice the protocol at home, unlike hands-on techniques, which are not easily accomplished without the therapist's continued guidance.

Overview

The exercise addresses two variants of FA: (1) breath-holding, which causes some clients to "mouth" words without transglottal airflow; and (2) hypercompressive laryngeal posture, resulting in intermittent high-pitched squeaking or strained whisper. The exercise first focuses on the stabilization of airflow through trans-nasal inspiration and pursed-lip expiration. It then facilitates transition from the voiceless flow of /s/ to the voiced airflow of /z/, under the masking of the therapist's modeling. Once this is accomplished, the therapist moves on to a resonating/m/, continuously voiced syllables, and counting.

The Exercise

1. Breathe in, allowing your abdomen to soften and expand, as though you were drawing in air into your belly. Breathe out through pursed (but not overly tensed) lips. Your cheeks should relax and inflate with the elevated breath pressure. If you experience difficulty breathing in and out in this relaxed fashion, try bubbling water in a cup by blowing through a straw, or gargling (which may elicit voicing).

2. Sustain an "ssss" sound for as long as you comfortably can. Make sure that you keep your lips and tongue free from tension as you produce the sound.

3. After you have achieved success in sustaining a tension-free "sss" sound, shift to a "zzzz" sound.

4. Allow the therapist to first sustain a "zzz" and then join in on the held sound.

5. Follow the therapist's model and substitute an "mmm" sound (hum) for the "zzz."

6. Continue to follow the therapist's model and slowly open your lips from the hum to a "moo" sound, as follows: "mmoom-moommoo." Make sure to match your therapist's rate.

7. Once you have achieved success with these sounds, follow your therapist's model and try to chant the following: "zoom-zoom-zoom" . . . "zoomba-zoomba-zoomba" . . . "zoo-one-zoo-one-zoo-one" . . . "zoo-one-two-zoo-one-two". . . "one-two-three-four-five" . . . "one-two-three-four-five (breath) six-seven-eight-nine-ten, etc."

8. Speak "one-two-three-four-five" and keep the sound continuous through the words. Keep your pitch in the same approximate range as your chant.

The therapist should help guide the client as to when the voiceless to voiced transition should occur. Both consonants should sound simultaneously for the second half of the utterance. Clients may have a tendency to stop during the unvoiced to voiced sibilant transition, in which case the therapist should provide a model loud enough to mask the client's production, in order to help the client begin voicing, and then decreasing the loudness of the modeling until the client's sound is dominant. The "chanted" /z/ will need to be pitched; I prefer Ab3 to Bb3 with adult females but this may vary, and if the client spontaneously jumps to a higher pitch while phonating, allow it to occur. Throughout all steps of this exercise, the therapist should fade the model as the client gains the ability to produce the target sound well.

Increase task difficulty by counting to 30 with breaths after every five numbers.

Gradually, phase more natural speech prosody into the number sequence (but try and keep words connected by sound rather than silence). Progress to other closed set lists such as days of week or months of the year using natural word separation. Graduated sentence lists are useful at this point as they provide a final transition to spontaneous conversation. Provide the client with a list of these steps so he or she can repeat the sequence at home should FA start to recur.

Cough or Throat-Clear
Phonation for Puberphonia

Edwin Yiu

Purpose

■ To lower falsetto-like pitch to normal male pitch range.

Origin

This exercise has been used widely by many therapists when working with postpubescent males who present with an abnormally high mean speaking pitch level.

Overview

Many therapists believe that one factor contributing to puberphonia is excessive laryngeal tension and habitual use of incoordinated laryngeal muscle activity. In these cases, the gentle cough or throat-clear can be produced sometimes using a normal pitch level, perhaps because it is a vegetative function and therefore not as susceptible to learned motor patterns.

Caution: It is commonly believed that frequent coughing and throat-clearing may be phonotraumatic. Therefore, it is essential that the client produce the cough or throat-clear in a gentle and slightly breathy manner, using good speech-breathing support. If the client is unable to produce the cough or throat-clear in a manner that is free of tension, this exercise should be abandoned.

The Exercise

1. Using good speech-breathing support, produce a soft and gentle cough /ʔha/ or throat-clear, listening for the low pitch of the vowel that may naturally occur toward the end of the cough or throat-clear. Repeat up to five times, taking a sip of water in between each gentle cough or throat-clear, until the low-normal pitch is clearly perceived. Make sure to take time in between each repetition to sip water, release tension in the upper torso, neck, and jaw, and replenish breath. If low-normal pitch is not produced after five attempts, abandon the exercise.

2. Produce the soft and gentle cough or throat-clear, slightly prolonging the vowel at a low pitch for one to two beats. Repeat

up to five times, taking a sip of water in between each repetition and pausing to release any buildup of tension and to replenish the breath.

3. After producing the cough or throat-clear and slightly prolonged vowel, close the lips to add a hum at the end of the maneuver, in the same low pitch as the vowel. The vowel should transition smoothly and continuously into the hum, with no break in airflow or voicing. Repeat up to five times, taking a sip of water in between each repetition and pausing to release any buildup of tension and replenish the breath.

4. Fade the cough or throat-clear, producing only the vowel (the end of the cough or throat-clear) at the low pitch, finishing up with the closed lips to form the hum. Repeat until accuracy is achieved consistently.

5. Fade out the vowel, producing only the hum /m/ at the new low pitch. Then, use the Hong Kong Humming exercise (Chapter 5) to shape the hum into speech.

Hiding Vocal Tremor

Julie Barkmeier-Kraemer

Purpose

■ To reduce the prominence of vocal tremor during speaking.

Origin

Shaping speech to hide vocal tremor during conversation by shortening the average duration of voicing is based on the premise that vocal tremor is easier to perceive during sustained phonation. In addition, individuals with vocal tremor tend to slow their rate of speech and prolong their speech sounds as vocal tremor worsens. Given that vocal tremor occurs at relatively slow rates (e.g., 4 to 12 Hz), transitions in speech sounds can be used to reduce the opportunity for listeners to hear voice modulations during conversation. This approach has been successfully taught to several individuals with vocal tremor. However, those with difficulty voluntarily producing a "staccato-like voice" may have more difficulty successfully shortening voicing duration during conversation.

Overview

Shortened voicing duration in conversation is achieved in a progressive manner, beginning with speech stimuli that facilitate easy voice onset combined with shortened, or staccato-like vowel production. Once individuals successfully produce shortened vowels, speech stimuli are used with voiceless speech sounds, followed by sentences composed of all-voiced speech sounds. It is not necessary to produce staccato-like speaking for this method to "hide" vocal tremor. Use of an exaggerated staccato speaking style in the training phases is helpful, but should be modified to fit the individual's speaking style. As progression into carryover activities occurs, clients should personalize their speaking style while maintaining their ability to shorten voicing duration. Other strategies that are helpful in achieving shortened voicing duration include the strategic insertion of pauses and increasing speaking rate to approximately five syllables per second.

Note: Individuals diagnosed with vocal tremor who exhibit severe vocal tremor in sustained phonation, voiceless-loaded sentences, and voice-loaded sentences, or who cannot purposely reduce their voicing duration during instruction to produce staccato-like speech, may not find this strategy helpful. For those individuals who fail to effectively shorten voicing duration using this exercise, producing increased breathiness during speaking appears to be a helpful alternative strategy.

The Exercises

1. Say each of the following words with an audible "h" sound followed by the shortest vowel sound you can produce (i.e., easy voice onset plus shortened vowel duration).

   a. He
   b. Who
   c. Hoe
   d. Hey
   e. Huh
   f. Ha

2. Say each of the following words with easy onset of the vowels, making sure to keep the duration of the vowel short, and then finish the word with a voiceless consonant. Using a staccato style of speaking may help.

   a. Half
   b. Hook
   c. Hoot
   d. Hoof
   e. Hip
   f. Hut
   g. Hate
   h. Hoop
   i. Hit
   j. Hat
   k. Hope
   l. Huff

3. Say each of the following two-syllable words keeping the same pattern of producing an audible "h" sound and shortened voicing within the word. Try to maintain the staccato style by saying the word at a faster rate.

   a. Happy
   b. Hippy
   c. Heater
   d. Hiccup
   e. Hockey
   f. Hanky
   g. Hooper
   h. Haughty
   i. Horses
   j. Husky
   k. Holster
   l. Hobo
   m. Handy
   n. Healer
   o. Hammer
   p. Henhouse
   q. Hundred
   r. Hailstorm
   s. Headache
   t. Hero

4. Expand the method above to phrases (using pauses sometimes helps with these):

   a. Help with hiccups
   b. Horses with hooves
   c. Who had a hammer?
   d. Halfway to heaven
   e. Healing with hugs
   f. Heat the henhouse
   g. He has a hero
   h. Howling hounds
   i. Hopeful hippy
   j. Hurt with hate
   k. He had hope
   l. His hit the hill

5. Expand to sentences loaded with voiceless sounds:

   a. She keeps a clean house.
   b. Sue saw a fellow fan.
   c. He saw a stellar hockey match.
   d. She took the package.
   e. The boat tipped to and fro.
   f. Chickens eat corn and seeds.
   g. Tell her about the party.
   h. Could you pick a peck of pepper?
   i. Some fish swim with turtles.
   j. Peter threw the football.

6. Practice using shortened voicing duration in single syllable words that are all voiced:

   a. Am
   b. Egg
   c. End
   d. And
   e. Eel
   f. Own
   g. Room
   h. Ale
   i. Mean
   j. Man
   k. Moan
   l. New
   m. Nail
   n. Moon
   o. My
   p. Wean
   q. One
   r. When

7. Practice using shortened voicing duration (staccato-like speaking) and faster speaking rate with two-syllable all-voiced words:

   a. Many
   b. Meany
   c. Melon
   d. Mary
   e. Maybe
   f. Amble
   g. Again
   h. Abbey
   i. Arrow
   j. Never
   k. Bellow
   l. Reward
   m. Wonder
   n. Noodle
   o. Owner
   p. Weaver

8. Expand to phrases and sentences loaded with all-voiced speech sounds:

    a. Anyone is allowed

    b. Many more may know

    c. Andy lead the way

    d. When will Mary run?

    e. A million dollar dog

    f. Another day began

    g. Rise in the morning.

    h. Money made the man.

    i. Red wine may remain

    j. Nelly never knew the way in.

    k. May you always be well.

    l. My name was never known.

9. Expand to phrases and sentences with mixed speech sounds:

    a. Several more were on their way.

    b. I have several more where that came from.

    c. She was very persistent and therefore succeeded.

    d. Why was he always in the front of the class?

    e. Tell me more about your life.

    f. I wonder what tomorrow will bring.

    g. She has a way about her that makes me smile.

    h. He had a hundred hounds on that farm.

    i. Shall we make chocolate chip cookies for dessert?

    j. How can I help make the world a better place?

    k. A helping had is always appreciated at the park.

    l. Will you come by the party and bring a dish?

    m. I plan to paddle the canoe to the end of the stream.

10. Practice reading a paragraph selected from a newspaper or magazine. Break the paragraph into short phrases and strategically insert pauses at times when you need to replenish your air supply, or begin to have difficulty hiding the vocal tremor.

11. Practice shortened voicing duration strategies during five minutes of a conversation. During this time, concentrate on keeping voicing durations shorter, speaking at a faster rate, and pausing when you need to replenish your air supply, or begin to hear the vocal tremor.

Conversational Voice Therapy

Alison Behrman

The exercises are intended primarily for clients who engage frequently in group discussions, presentations, and one-on-one high-consequence conversations.

Conversation is the exchange of ideas. One premise of these exercises is that effective conversation is achieved through connection with individuals, even when speaking to a group (such as teaching a class or presenting an idea to a team). Consequently, the behavioral changes that are targeted in these exercises are motivated by improving the client's voice through more effective interpersonal connections.

A second premise is that authenticity promotes interpersonal connection. Clients may become resistant to vocal behavioral change when they think that the results will make them sound inauthentic (Behrman, Rutledge, Hembree, & Sheridan; 2008). However, in reality, the authentic self that most speakers *intend* to project, often, is not what is *actually* projected to the listener. Many speakers are not fully aware of the impressions that they make on their listeners: a gap may exist between the speaker's intention and the listener's impression, and it is the therapist's role to close that gap. Conversational voice therapy is designed to give speakers conscious control over selected behaviors, helping the speaker to display outwardly his or her inner concept of authentic self. Consequently, throughout the exercises, the therapist is encouraged to return often to the effect of the behavior changes on the overall impression the client is projecting to the listeners.

Purposes

- To promote healthy voice production, particularly when speaking in high-consequence conversations, group discussions, and presentations.
- To improve communicative effectiveness through increased connection between speakers and their listeners.

Origin

I have spent a number of years coaching executives in public speaking skills and conducting therapy for patients with voice disorders. In my mixed practice, I couldn't help but notice the voice quality improvements of many of my public speaking clients; in particular, decreased harshness and nasality, and increased oral resonance. Many of these same clients noted a similar improvement in their voices when they compared recordings of their presentations before and after coaching. I considered the possible reasons for the perceived vocal improvement. The coaching techniques, directly or indirectly, facilitated slower speech, greater movement of the articulators, greater breath support, and wider intonation contour. I hypothesized that these changes might well increase oral resonance and yield a more pleasing vocal quality. I began to explore the application of these techniques to my voice therapy patients. In particular, I targeted my patients whose occupational vocal demands required them to make group presentations (e.g., teachers) or one-on-one high-consequence conversations (e.g., counselors). The outcomes have been encouraging, and I hope you find them similarly useful.

Overview

Conversational voice therapy is composed of five exercises: pausing, visual connection, clear vowels, vocal variety, and physical connection, accompanied by frequent video analyses. Portions of these exercises are already part of many therapists' repertoires. The difference here is the focus upon enhancing the effectiveness of the speaker's communicative connection with the listener. The distinction is important because, I believe, it helps the speaker to naturally integrate these techniques into important and stressful communicative acts: the situations in which maintaining healthy voice use can be most difficult. Hence, the therapist is urged to engage the client frequently in discussion and provide feedback on the effect of the target behaviors on their communicative connection with their listeners.

The Exercises

It is recommended that pausing be addressed first. It is the most basic skill and a prerequisite for all additional skills. It is deceptively simple to describe, but quite challenging for most clients to integrate into conversation, particularly those clients who naturally use lots of filler words. The order in which the other exercises are presented to a given client may vary. The therapist is encouraged to combine different exercises after the client has achieved success with individual components.

Pausing

1. Start by pausing at every period, using an exaggerated pause of two full beats. All pauses are completely silent, with no fillers such as "um" or "and." Next, pause for two beats at all commas and periods. Initially, the pause will feel extraordinarily long. After you have achieved success using the exaggerated pause at all periods and commas, reduce the duration to one beat. Ultimately, the length of the pause will vary, and will be determined by the needs of the speaker and the listener.

2. Return to the exaggerated length pause and briefly inhale during each pause. Make sure not to inhale deeply, which is unnecessary and counterproductive. Do make sure to inhale by expanding the lower thorax/abdomen.

3. Identify a monologue or discussion topic in which you commonly engage at work, and use it to practice pausing.

4. Optional: You may want to try Physical Connection exercises 1 and 2 of at this point, to connect the verbal pause with a physical release of tension.

> Clients who are not familiar with diaphragmatic breathing, or who confuse speed of the inhalation with the volume of air, will likely benefit from attention to breathing exercises before attempting to connect the inhale with the pause. Use the term "inhale" rather than "breathe" during instruction. Otherwise, you risk having the client complete a full breathe cycle (inhale and exhale) during the pause, and then the client is left with insufficient air for the next utterance.

Visual Connection

1. Using low-content spontaneous conversation, look at your listener when speaking. If desired, glance away briefly during a pause and then return to look at your conversational partner when starting to speak again until eye contact becomes more comfortable for you. Resist the urge to glance away (at the floor, ceiling, or over your listener's shoulder) when speaking. It breaks the connection between you and your listener.

2. Prepare a one- to two-minute monologue. Direct your eye gaze to your first listener, and begin your monologue. When you

Eye gaze is best learned in a group, but most therapy is private. A solution is to set up the room with at least four seats distributed in a rough semicircle around the client. Sit in one of the seats. Direct the client to begin the monologue, establishing eye contact first with you as listener one. When you feel that the client has come to the end of a thought and is pausing, move to another seat. You are now listener two and the client should turn to establish a connection (eye contact) with you as a "new" listener. Continue on through the client's monologue, moving from one seat to another during pauses. Do not always move to an adjacent seat, so that the client can become accustomed to moving visually about the room to engage listeners in a random pattern.

come to the end of a thought group or two (often one or two sentences), pause and direct your gaze to another listener, and begin your next sentence. Continue in this fashion for all listeners. Make sure that you do not start to speak until you have connected visually with your listener, and do not look away until you have finished your sentence and you are in a silent pause. After the exercise, get feedback from your listeners about whether they felt connected to you by your eye gaze, or whether they needed longer eye gaze from you.

3. Repeat Step 2 above, but now direct each of your listeners to give you a "thumb's up" sign when they feel that you have connected strongly with them. Advise your listeners that they may give you this signal only after you have conclude a thought group (during a silent pause), and only if they feel you have connected authentically with them individually. As the speaker, you may move on to the next listener only after you have received the signal your current listener. If you have connected with each listener but have not finished your talk, then revisit individual listeners, but in a different gaze pattern. When you conclude this step, discuss with your listeners their impressions of you.

Clear Vowels

1. Say the following words and overenunciate the vowels. Select a mental image of the vowels (perhaps a large red balloon) and use that visualization to help you focus on the vowels.

you	debut	argue	youth
aura	macaw	auto	also
lie	riot	eyes	five
vow	how	kowtow	vowel
coal	show	only	Oreo
fate	okay	daily	eight

2. Read aloud some text provided by your therapist, but read *only* the vowels. You will not be intelligible and it will sound odd. For example, for the utterance "read this aloud," it would sound like "ee ih uh ow." Try to use the rhythm and syllable stress of the sentence that you would use if reading the sentence normally. Immediately after completing this step, re-read the text including all of the sounds (reading "normally") but try to continue to visualize the vowels and emphasize them.

3. For this step, use each of the following vowels in turn: ah (as in hot), oh (as in hoe), ee (as in heat), and oo (as in hoot). Start with the first vowel and insert it into the following nonsense

words, overenunciating the vowels. Then repeat the nonsense words, this time inserting the second vowel. Continue through all four vowels. (In the following list, the capital V represents the vowel to be inserted.)

cVdV   pVtV   sVlA   fVrV

4. Repeat exercise 3 above, but now place each nonsense word in the phrase:

I see a [nonsense word] by the house.

Focus on overenunciating the vowels, not only in the nonsense word, but also in the other words in the phrase. Once you have achieved success on this exercise, repeat it, but decrease the exaggeration of the vowels a little. The goal is to maintain the vowel overenunciation while restoring natural-sounding speech.

5. Now, starting with reading, pronounce the vowels clearly, as if speaking to someone from a different language background or who otherwise has difficulty understanding your words easily. Once this speaking style becomes comfortable while reading, practice clear vowels in simple conversation and then more complex discussion, and finally, with a topic in which you commonly engage at work.

Vocal Variety

1. Read aloud a passage with a "singsong" style (exaggerated vocal variety). It may be helpful to pretend that you are telling a story to young children. Alternatively, consider the analogy to move your pitch up and down "like a boat riding over big waves" or "like riding on a roller coaster." Make sure to use brief silent pauses at all punctuation.
2. Repeat Step 1 above, but decrease the singsong style by 20%. Continue to monitor your pausing during the exercise. With repeated readings, alter (upward or downward) the degree of vocal variety by specific percentages as directed by your therapist, until you obtain a natural-sounding but expressive voice.
3. Prepare a list of questions, from simple (Is it supposed to rain today?) to more complex (Why do you think most people get annoyed when someone is talking loudly on their cell phone in a public place?) Use exaggerated vocal variety while alternating roles as the questioner or responder with a conversational partner. Avoid using single-word responses.
4. Repeat Step 3 above, again decreasing singsong style by 20%, following the directions of Step 2 for continuing to adjust the amount of vocal variety.

5. With your conversational partner, make statements that elicit a contradictory or corrective response. For example, in the following exchange, the underlining shows the target words for greater pitch changes.

> SLP: "Joe is *my* friend."
>
> Client: "No, he's *not.* Joe is *my* friend. *Warren* is *your* friend."

Alternate roles with your conversational partner.

6. Identify a monologue or discussion topic in which you commonly engage at work. Think about the words and ideas that you want to emphasize. Then, give the monologue to, or engage in discussion with, your therapist, using exaggerated vocal variety to emphasize the words and ideas that you have previously identified. (It may be helpful to write out some of the text beforehand in order to identify the desired emphasis. However, it is important that you then put it away, and speak spontaneously, recognizing that the specific words you use will change.)

Physical Connection

1. Begin by practicing the neutral stance. Stand with your weight equally distributed on both legs, feet approximately hip width apart. Your spine is elongated and you are standing tall, chin level with the floor, shoulders relaxed downward, arms hanging at the sides. Remember to breathe! It may be helpful to visualize one string attached to your sternum and a second string to the crown of your head, each connected to the ceiling and pulling you upward gently. Experience this position for a few beats and report on the experience to your therapist. This posture may feel uncomfortable initially. This stance is the neutral position. Walk a few steps and then return to neutral, reach up as though putting something on a top shelf, and return to neutral, bend down, and then return to neutral.

2. Using low-content dialogue, such as a "how-to" explanation, engage in dialogue with your therapist, and return to the neutral stance during each pause. Take the time to use an exaggerated pause so that you have the time to fully regain your neutral stance.

3. Prepare a short (1-minute) monologue on a topic with which you are familiar and comfortable. Begin in the neutral position, keeping the lower half of your body immobile (the feet do not move) throughout the exercise. The rationale for this restriction is that connection with the listener is not achieved through the lower body. Typically, when someone uses a lot of movement in the lower body (such as random pacing or foot movements), it is distracting to both the listener and the

---

The client may become constrained in movement or vocal energy during this exercise, because of the focus upon the neutral stance during the pause. For the moment, ignore that problem: the next step will address it. The critical learning in this exercise is that the pause now becomes a full body release of tension, not just a verbal pause.

speaker, and can result in postural imbalance and, we hypothesize, increased tension.

4. Present the monologue to your therapist, maintaining throughout the talk the energy level directed by your therapist. Initially, exaggerate each pause, using two beats, and return to neutral stance each time.

5. When you have achieved 80% accuracy with step 4, repeat it, decreasing the pause and neutral stance duration to one beat each time.

6. When you have achieved 80% accuracy with Step 5, repeat it once more, this time varying the duration of the pause and the neutral stance to meet the needs of your listener.

7. Repeat Steps 3 through 6, but this time incorporating Visual Connection exercise 2, (engaging more than one listener with eye contact). Make sure to return to the neutral position during each pause

8. Proceed through Steps 1 through 7 above, but this time from a seated position. The neutral position in the chair requires at least one foot completely on the ground (so one leg may be crossed). You should be sitting all the way back in the chair with your back comfortably resting on the back of the chair. You arms are resting on the armrests, or at rest in your lap, but your hands are not clasped together and your arms are not crossed on the chest. (Caution with swivel chairs—no swiveling!)

9. Optional. Engage your listener in conversation. Reach out to with the core by leaning forward slightly toward your listener (bend a bit at the waist) to emphasize a point intermittently. Alternatively, or additionally, produce a monologue to practice this behavior. Reaching out with the core is particularly important if you tend to jut out your chin (head) only when speaking.

> Ask your client "How much energy do you usually exhibit when you talk, with 1 being no energy and 10 being over-the-top energy?" If you have observed that your client is tight and locked in with tension, then ask the client to move up the energy scale by 5 points. If you have observed that your client has a lot of energy, perhaps even tense energy, direct the client to give the monologue at his or her self-rated point on the energy scale.

> Many clients require considerable coaching to switch between high energy during speaking and then neutral, relaxed stance (with accompanying inhale during the pause). This step is important for achieving balance between relaxed body and natural energy, and will be quite difficult for many clients to achieve initially. When the client is ready to use a variable length pause and accompanying neutral stance, discuss first what conditions might encourage longer or shorter pauses. For example, the pause should be longer to emphasize a point or to start a new segment of information, and shorter for a quick inhale or to continue with an idea.

Video Analysis

Video analysis is particularly helpful in facilitating discussion on the effect of the target behavior changes on the overall impression the client is projecting to the listeners.

1. At the first therapy session, obtain a baseline video. Record one and a half to two minutes of a client monologue. Ideally, the client should select a topic commonly addressed at work, one on which the client is comfortable and knowledgeable speaking. Less desirable, but feasible, is to describe a recent trip, hobby or other topic on which the client can talk for the required time.
   a. View the video with the client silently. Then, ask questions to generate introspection on the part of the client, such as: "What surprises you about how you look and/or sound?"; "If you were a stranger watching the video, what impressions

would you have about the speaker?"; and "What do you like and dislike about the impression you are portraying?"

b. Then, provide your assessment. It is important that your assessment focuses upon the interpersonal connection the client is achieving. Link the assessment to: (1) the client's self-impressions generated in (a) above; (2) the five dimensions of pausing, visual and physical connections, vowel clarity, vocal variety, and grounding; and (3) the connection to vocal improvement.

2. At most subsequent therapy sessions, video record short speaking segments (one minute or less) to provide feedback to demonstrate: (1) improvement; (2) error in the client's perception; and (3) introduction of a new behavior. Engage your client in introspective dialogue with question, including: What does this behavior (the newly demonstrated target behavior) do for your listener and your connection with the listener? What does it do for your voice?

3. On a regular basis, require the client video him/herself in select conversational/presentational encounters. Review and analyze these videos during subsequent therapy sessions.

GLOSSARY

Arpeggio: a musical term describing playing the notes of a chord in succession (one after the other) rather than simultaneously.

Breath support: *see* Speech-breathing support.

Breathy phonation: voice production which uses excessive airflow, yielding a voice quality that is often soft or weak-sounding.

Chanting: using a legato or linked style of speaking on a monopitch.

Crescendo: gradual increase in loudness level.

Diminuendo: gradual decrease in loudness level.

Falsetto register: occupies the frequencies above modal register. This register is most easily recognized in the male voice at a very high pitch.

Flow phonation: a manner of voice production that yields the highest ratio between output sound pressure level and input subglottal pressure.

Glissando: smoothly produced vocal glide upward or downward in pitch.

Glottal fry: a mode of phonation in which the fundamental frequency is quite low, approximately 35 Hz to 50 Hz, in both men and women. Also called *pulse register*.

Legato: producing sounds in a smoothly gliding manner; maintaining voicing across word boundaries, and thus decreasing voice onsets and offsets. Also called linking or continuous phonation. Contrast with *staccato*.

Messa di voce: a musical technique involving a slow crescendo (increasing loudness) followed smoothly by a slow decrescendo (decreasing loudness).

Modal register: the register within which most speech occurs. The span of frequencies in modal register is approximately 90 to 450 Hz for men and 150 to 520 Hz for women.

Phonotrauma: voice use patterns leading to traumatic tissue changes of the vocal folds.

Pressed phonation: an inefficient manner of voice production in which a high level of subglottal pressure is combined with high adductory force of the vocal folds, yielding low airflow.

Proprioception: a sense of the position of one's body in space.

Pulse register: *see* Glottal fry.

Register: a series of consecutive values of fundamental frequencies of approximately equivalent vocal quality. Register refers to particular modes of vibration of the vocal folds, including *glottal fry* (pulse), *modal*, and *falsetto*.

Resonance: a large increase in the amplitude of a vibration when a force is applied at a natural frequency of an object or medium. In voice therapy, frequently implies a sensation of dominance of acoustic energy in the front of the mouth and face, achieved through manipulation of the position of the vocal tract and articulators, to achieve a pleasant-sounding voice that is heard easily and produced with minimal effort.

Speech-breathing support: the regulation of breathing for voice and speech production.

Staccato: producing sounds of very short duration; a rapid, clipped manner of articulating, using frequent voice onsets and offsets. Contrast with *legato*.

REFERENCES

Adler, R. K., Hirsch, S., & Mordaunt, M. (2006). *Voice and communication therapy for the transgender/transsexual client: A comprehensive clinical guide*. San Diego, CA: Plural.

Andrews, M. (2002). *Voice treatment for children and adolescents*. Clifton Park, NY: Singular-Thomson Learning.

Aronson, A. E. (1981). *Clinical voice disorders: An interdisciplinary approach* (3rd ed.). New York, NY: Thieme-Stratton.

Behlau, M. (1994). *Técnicas de reabilitação vocal*. São Paulo, Brazil: CEV.

Behrman, A. (2006). Facilitating behavioral change in voice therapy: The relevance of motivational interviewing. *American Journal of Speech-Language Pathology, 15*, 1-11.

Boies, L. R., Hilger, J. A., & Priest, R. E. (1964). *Fundamentals of otolaryngology*. Philadelphia, PA: W. B. Saunders.

Boone, D. R. (2004). *The voice and voice therapy* (8th ed.). Boston, MA: Allyn & Bacon.

Boone, D. R., & McFarlane, S. C. (1999). *The voice and voice therapy* (7th ed.) Boston, MA: Pearson Education.

Briess, B. (1957). Voice therapy- part 1: Identification of specific laryngeal muscle dysfunction by voice testing. *Archives of Otolaryngology, 66*, 61-69.

Briess, B. (1959). Voice therapy- part II: Essential treatment phases of laryngeal muscle dysfunction. *Archives of Otolaryngology, 69*, 61-69.

Carroll, L. M. (2000). Application of singing techniques for the treatment of dysphonia. *Otolaryngologic Clinics of North America, 33*(5), 1003-1015.

Casteel, R., & Stone Jr., R. (1983). In M. Filter (Ed.), *Phonatory voice disorders in children*. Springfield, IL: Charles C. Thomas.

Christopher, K. L., Wood, R. P. 2nd., Eckert, R. C., Blager, F. B., Raney, R. A., & Souhrada, J. F. (1983). Vocal-cord dysfunction presenting as asthma. *New England Journal of Medicine, 308*, 1566-1570.

Colton, R. H., Casper, J. K., & Leonard, R. (2006). *Understanding voice problems: A physiological perspective for diagnosis and treatment* (3rd ed.). Philadelphia, PA: Lippincott Williams & Wilkins.

DeJonckere, P. H. (1998). Effect of louder voicing on acoustical measurements in dysphonic patients. *Logopedics, Phoniatrics, Vocology, 23*, 79-84.

DeJonckere, P. H., & Lebacq, J. (2001). Plasticity of voice quality: A prognostic factor for outcome of voice therapy? *Journal of Voice, 15*, 251-256.

DeJonckere, P. H., & Wieneke, G. G. (2001). Basic elements in voice therapy. In *Occupational voice, care and cure* (pp. 155-163). The Hague, Netherlands: Kugler.

Froeschels, E. (1952). Chewing method as therapy: A discussion with some philosophical conclusions. *A.M.A. Archives of Otolaryngology, 56*, 427-434.

Froeschels, E., Kastein, S., & Weiss, D.A.(1955). A method of therapy for paralytic conditions of the mechanisms of phonation, respiration, and glutination. *Journal of Speech and Hearing Disorders, 20*, 365-370.

Garber, C. E., Blissmer, B., Deschenes, M. R., Franklin, B. A., Lamonte, M. J., Lee, I. M., . . . Swain, D. P. (2011). American College of Sports Medicine position stand. Quantity and quality of exercise for developing and maintaining cardiorespiratory, musculoskeletal, and neuromotor fitness in apparently healthy adults: Guidance for prescribing exercise. *Medicine Science Sports Exercise, 43*, 1334-1359.

Gauffin, J., & Sundberg, J. (1989). Spectral correlates of glottal voice source waveform characteristics. *Journal of Speech and Hearing Research, 32*, 556-565.

Gleason, E. B. (1928). *A manual of diseases of the nose, throat and ear*. Bristol, UK: John Wright and Sons Ltd.

Harris, T., Harris, S., Rubin, J. S., & Howard, D. M. (1998). *The voice clinic handbook*. London, UK: Whurr.

Heuer, R. J., Sataloff, R.T., Emerich, K., Rulnick, R., Baroody, M., Spiegel, J.R., et al. (1997). Unilateral recurrent laryngeal nerve paralysis: the importance of "preoperative" voice therapy. *Journal of Voice, 11*, 88-94.

Laukkanen, A.M. (1992). About the so-called "resonance tubes" used in Finnish voice training practice. *Scandinavian Journal of Logopedics and Phoniatrics, 17,* 151–161.

Laukkanen, A-M., Lindholm, P., & Vilkman, E. (1995). Phonation into a tube as a voice training method. Acoustic and physiologic observations. *Folia Phoniatrica et Logopaedica, 47,* 331–338.

Lessac, A. (1960*). The use and training of the human voice* (3rd ed.). New York, NY: McGraw-Hill.

Linklater, K. (1976). *Freeing the natural voice.* New York, NY: Drama Books.

Lyle, H. (2012). *Vocal yoga: The joy of singing, breathing and sounding.* Pacific Palisades, CA: Bluecat Music and Publishing.

Martens, J. W., Versnel, H., & DeJonckere, P. H. (2007). The effect of visible speech in the perceptual rating of pathological voices. *Archives of Otolaryngology-Head and Neck Surgery, 133,* 178–185.

Melov, S., Tarnopolsky, M. A., Beckman, K., Felkey, K., & Hubbard, A. (2007). Resistance exercise reverses aging in human skeletal muscle. *PLoS One, 2*(5), e465.

Miller, W. R., & Rollnick, S. (2002). *Motivational interviewing: Preparing people for change* (2nd ed.). New York, NY: Guilford Press.

Miriam-Webster's collegiate dictionary. (2004). (10th ed.). New York, NY: Collegiate.

Moncur, J. P., & Brackett, I. P. (1974). *Modifying vocal behavior.* New York, NY: Harper and Row.

Peterson, M. D., Rhea, M. R., Sen, A., & Gordon, P. M. (2010). Resistance exercise for muscular strength in older adults: A meta-analysis. *Ageing Research Reviews, 9,* 226–237.

Prochaska, J. O., Norcross, J. C., & DiClemente, C. C. (1994). *Changing for good: The revolutionary program that explains the six stages of change and teaches you how to free yourself from bad habits.* New York, NY: W. Morrow.

Ramig, L. O., Countryman, S., Thompson, L. L., & Horii, Y. (1995). Comparison of two forms of intensive speech treatment for Parkinson disease. *Journal of Speech, Language, Hearing Research, 38,* 1232–1251.

Ramig, L. O., Fox, C., & Sapir, S. (2004). Parkinson's disease: Speech and voice disorders and their treatment with the Lee Silverman Voice Treatment. *Seminars in Speech and Language. 25,* 169–180.

Riley, W. D., Korovin, G. S., & Gould, W. J. *Directed energy in vocal technique: A preliminary study of clinical application.* Presented at The Voice Foundation Symposium: Care of the Professional Voice, Philadelphia, PA, June 7, 1990.

Rollnick, S., Mason, P., & Butler, C. (1999). *Health behavior change: A guide for practitioners.* London, UK: Churchill Livingstone.

Roy, N., Bless, D. M., Heisey, D., & Ford, C. N.(1997). Manual circumlaryngeal therapy for functional dysphonia: An evaluation of short- and long-term treatment outcomes. *Journal of Voice, 11,* 321–331.

Sataloff, R. T., Baroody, M. E., Emerich, K. A., & Carroll, L. M. (2005). The singing voice specialist. In R. T. Sataloff. *Professional voice: The science and art of clinical care* (p. 1037). San Diego, CA: Plural.

Schmidt, R. A., & Lee, T. D. (2011). *Motor control and learning: A behavioral emphasis* (5th ed.). Champaign, IL: Human Kinetics.

Sihvo, M., & Denizoglu, I. (2007). *Lax VoxR: Voice therapy technique.* Izmir, Turkey: AD .

Stemple, J. (2000). *Clinical voice pathology: Theory and management* (3rd ed). Clifton Park, NY: Delmar-Thomson Learning.

Stemple, J. C., Lee, L., D'Amico, B., & Pickup, B. (1994). Efficacy of vocal function exercises as a method of improving voice production. *Journal of Voice, 8,* 271–278.

Story, B. H., Titze, I. R., & Hoffman, E. A. (1996). Vocal tract area functions from magnetic resonance imaging. *Journal of the Acoustical Society of America, 100,* 537–554.

Titze, I. (2006). Voice training and therapy with a semi-occluded vocal tract: Rationale and scientific underpinnings. *Journal of Speech, Language, and Hearing Research, 49,* 448–459.

Titze, I. R. (2000). Phonation into a straw as a voice building exercise. *Journal of Singing, 57,* 27–28.

Turecki, S. (2000) *The difficult child* (2nd ed). New York, NY: Bantam.

Verdolini, K. (1999). *A guide to vocology.* Iowa City, IA: National Center of Speech and Voice.

Verdolini, K., Druker, D. G., Palmer, P. M., & Samawi, H. (1998). Laryngeal adduction in resonant voice. *Journal of Voice, 12,* 315–327.

Yamaguchi, H., Yotsukura, Y., Sata, H., Watanabe, Y., Hirose, H., Kobayashi, N., et al. (1993). Pushing exercise program to correct glottal incompetence. *Journal of Voice, 7,* 250–256.

INDEX